What People Are Saying About
The New Prescription

"*The New Prescription* contains hundreds of practical tips for improving the medical care you receive while saving thousands of dollars each year. Dr. Haines's approach puts you in the driver's seat, and this book provides a reliable 'navigator' to guide you through our complex and confusing medical 'system.'"

—Art Ulene, M.D., health educator
and former "family doctor" on NBC's *Today*

"Dr. Haines highlights some of the key problems that people face—how to get the best possible medical care without unnecessary time, expense, and procedures. This is an excellent guide and one that will save readers not only money, but much suffering."

—Julie Silver, M.D., assistant professor at
Harvard Medical School and author of
several award-winning health books, including
*What Helped Get Me Through:
Cancer Survivors Share Wisdom and Hope*

"If health care in the twenty-first century dictates that patients be 'informed healthcare consumers' in the physician-patient relationship, then Dr. Cynthia Haines has the right prescription for their success. For the first time in history, patients are bombarded with a constant, always-on, twenty-four-hour avalanche of information regarding health care. Even before we begin to make sense of it all, it helps to know how to navigate that sea of information. Dr. Haines provides the blueprint for that understanding in simple to understand but compelling thoughts. Ultimately, patients are responsible for the choices they make in this new reality of healthcare delivery. Dr. Haines's points succinctly complement other tools at the patient-as-healthcare-consumers' disposal to personalize health care and make it work for them. I wish she was my primary-care doctor."

—Michael Douglas, M.D., MBA, editor/proprietor of the
Doctor Pundit health-care policy blog

"Dr. Haines knows that effective communication is the cornerstone of optimal health care. Here, she offers her insights to help not just consumers of health care, but the providers of it as well."

—Teresa Knight, M.D., CEO of Women's
Health Specialists of Saint Louis

"Through the savvy, smart tips of Dr. Cindy Haines, you can gain a sense of empowerment now, before visiting another doctor's office or any hospital. You can be an insider in your own health care with her guidance."

—John La Puma, M.D., author of *ChefMD's
Big Book of Culinary Medicine* and host of the
PBS special Eat and Cook Healthy with Dr. John La Puma

"We live in a society where being unhealthy is the prerequisite for getting sound health care. Through a narrative of simple examples that confront us every day as individuals, parents, and caretakers of our family and friends, Dr. Cynthia Haines challenges us to not be the patient, but to be a wise consumer of healthcare options. The book is a preface to the patient engagement that is essential for reforming our healthcare system. Dr. Haines's book lays out in simple ways the basic truths we must acknowledge in our journey to becoming a healthy society. It helps us think clearly as we take charge of our most precious asset—our health—without the prejudice of consumerism that has been ingrained in our thinking when it comes to health care for us as individuals and our families. I call this book the starting point for Consumer Empowerment in Healthcare Improvement."

—Tom M. Gomez, founder and
executive director of Transformations at the Edge

"What every patient needs to understand how to get the most out of our healthcare system . . . or how to need it less. This complex healthcare system can be very confusing for most of us, no matter how good our insurance is. *The New Prescription* will help the reader learn to use the system without being harmed."

—David Schneider, M.D., professor and chairman of the
Department of Family and Community Medicine at Saint
Louis University School of Medicine

"Dr. Cindy Haines takes a sensible approach to explain the health-care dilemma we are faced with in the United States today. The material provided in her book is presented in a reader-friendly format that is chock-full of informational nuggets. This book offers concrete steps the reader can follow to get the maximum benefit from each encounter with the healthcare system, and that can make a positive impact on their health today."

—Tim Peters, president of MedActionPlan.com, LLC

"Dr. Cindy Haines gives us readers the greatest gift possible with her book *The New Prescription* . . . She lays out a step-by-step guide that empowers us to become "health seekers" rather than passive, dependent patients in an overburdened healthcare system. As a career mother of a large family, I am so thankful to have this clear blueprint about how to truly navigate the healthcare system and take control of my family's health care."

—Anne Wells, founder of UNITE the World with Africa and author of *Raising Babies and Raising Kids in St. Louis*

"With the complexity of healthcare decisions facing consumers, Dr. Haines offers practical insights and resourceful alternatives for patients and families who are seeking the best medical care for their loved ones. Her keen professional insight is relayed in an appealing, easily accessible format."

—Karen Lee Bechert, M.D., MPH, Harvard-trained geriatrician, public health worker, consumer health educator, and founder of MD Kiosk Health Channel

"Dr. Haines provides an invaluable insider's perspective and serves as a trusted guide to achieving health in a sometimes treacherous healthcare system."

—Stephen Brunton, M.D., adjunct clinical professor, Department of Family Medicine at University of North Carolina, Chapel Hill, and executive vice president for education at Primary Care Education Consortium

"This book is like having a personal physician guide you through an often confusing medical system. Lots of good advice on how to stay healthy, which is even more valuable. Highly recommended."

—Charles O. Elson, M.D., professor of medicine
at University of Alabama at Birmingham

"As a family physician, I recommend Dr. Cindy Haines's book. It is a great resource for patients to help themselves obtain the good health and good medical care that they desire in a system that can be confusing and hard to navigate. I highly recommend this book."

—Caroline Rudnick, M.D., Ph.D., president of
the St. Louis Academy of Family Physicians

"A book like this is a necessary guide in a time when the health-care system is undergoing enormous change. It gives readers and consumers a road map on how to maximize their health as they increasingly have to bear the costs of their care. Dr. Haines's book offers a really terrific, no-nonsense, practical look at health care and how to navigate the system from someone who has seen it from all points of view. Knowing how the system really works can work to your benefit. *The New Prescription* strips away the mystery of it all."

—Brett Johnson, president and executive
editor of OneMedPlace

The New Prescription:

How to Get the Best Health Care in a Broken System

CYNTHIA HAINES, M.D.
with ERIC METCALF, M.P.H.

Health Communications, Inc.
Deerfield Beach, Florida

www.hcibooks.com

Library of Congress Cataloging-in-Publication Data

Haines, Cynthia.
   The new prescription : how to get the best health care in a broken
system / Cynthia Haines with Eric Metcalf.
      p.   cm.
   Includes bibliographical references.
   ISBN-13: 978-0-7573-1555-8
   ISBN-10: 0-7573-1555-0
   ISBN-13: 978-0-7573-9186-6 (ebook)
   ISBN-10: 0-7573-9186-9 (ebook)
   1. Medical care—United States—Popular works. I. Metcalf, Eric.
II. Title
RA395.A3H335 2011
362.1—dc22
                                                          2010051678

Publisher: Health Communications, Inc.
            3201 S.W. 15th Street
            Deerfield Beach, FL 33442–8190

Cover design by Justin Rotkowitz
Interior design and formatting by Lawna Patterson Oldfield

*This book is dedicated to
my husband and my children:
I am, because of you.*

Contents

Acknowledgments

This book would never have happened without the vision, hard work, and dedication of several people.

I would like to begin by thanking my coauthor, Eric, for his enduring devotion to this book as well as to the craft of writing. You are a gifted communicator who makes the magic that can come from well-crafted writing happen time and time again.

The other critical players in this process are numerous. Thank you to our literary agent, Linda Konner, of the Linda Konner Literary Agency in New York City; Linda, thank you for seeing the potential in our ideas and for taking us on and finding our book a home. To that end, infinite thanks to our faithful editor at HCI Books, Inc., Allison Janse, who believed in the message of our book and made my dream of becoming a published author a reality.

Thank you to all the editors and other staff at HCI Books, Inc., who nipped, tucked, and packaged our book to near perfection (I know, I know . . . no subjectivity here at all on my part!). Specifically, I'd like to thank Nicole Haye for her genius of new media and generosity in sharing it with me.

I'd also like to take this opportunity to express my gratitude to several other people who have helped me become a better writer, editor, communicator—and just a better person—along the way:

To the entire gang at HealthDay, especially Dan McKillen, who is about as kindred of a thinker as I have ever come across (must be that County Cork connection); Barry Hoffman, who will always remain editor in chief in my heart—the big voice with an even bigger heart who took a chance on a relatively unknown midwesterner and always believed in me; George Giokas, a trusted colleague and even more trusted friend who not only always gets the job done but also never forgets how much kindness matters.

And last, but certainly not least, I thank my family and friends for bringing love, light, and joy into my life every day. To my husband, Will, who also happens to be the best friend anyone could ever hope for (in addition to being an amazing father and the very essence of noble), and my children, Isabella Mary and William Dennison: Thank you for letting me be me . . . and loving me anyway! You are the sun around which my world turns.

I also want to thank the rest of my family, who have boundless, unconditional love for me that I feel and know even if we may not say it nearly enough. Mom and Dad, thank you for being my first and most frequent supporters. You taught me that as long as I think I can, I can. To Rich and Mary, thank you for giving me the most precious gift anyone could—a gift cherished more than words could possibly detail. To the rest of my beloved family and friends: I am amazed by what a smart and truly beautiful group you are. Not only do you (without fail) support me, you also reliably lift me up. I always know where to turn—to celebrate, commiserate, and/or laugh it off. Much love right back 'atcha.

Eric would like to thank his parents and the rest of his family for all their support and encouragement over the years and specifically during this project. He'd also like to mention his son, Milo, who will enjoy seeing his name in a book.

Introduction

*P*eople use the following call for wisdom as a way to guide many of their decisions, and it may help you attain better results from a healthcare system that often provides poor outcomes at a high cost:

> *". . . grant me the serenity to accept the things*
> *I cannot change; courage to change the things I can;*
> *and the wisdom to know the difference."*

If you have a compelling need to control your circumstances like I do, you know that the need for control can lead to a great deal of suffering. I definitely have the so-called type A personality. Those who know me have described me as intense, driven, and achieving. This nature is both a blessing and a curse. I get a lot done, but I also tend to have a hard time letting go. However, we *must* know when it's time to take action, and we must know when it's time to let go of the situation and trust that it will work out.

This book is about getting what you really want: better health on your own terms. Learning more about our healthcare system and how best to navigate it in its current form is critical for getting there. This involves learning how to work more effectively and efficiently within our healthcare system, as well as learning how to rely on it *less*.

These days, a lot of Americans seem to want to use the healthcare system to control their health as thoroughly as possible. Many people have come to see health care as the end-all solution to a life free of illness and discomfort. It's not. The healthcare system *can* accomplish great results. But it simply cannot change certain things. A lifetime of poor lifestyle decisions can't be undone by a trip to the doctor's office or emergency room, for example.

On the other hand, a lot of people don't realize that they have great power to change their own health. The way they eat, the way they use their bodies, and the way they maintain their outlook on the world can often do much more to maintain their health and prevent disease than the healthcare system can.

And harnessing the power of our healthcare resources to do the most good requires accepting the problems that surgery and medications can't change, having the courage to work on the problems that we can change on our own, and gaining the wisdom to know the difference between the two.

I hope this book helps you get there.

Some people are dancers, born to dance. Others are born to cook and subsequently become chefs. I communicate. When I was interviewing for entrance into medical school, one of the faculty remarked on my essay, saying that he thought I should reconsider my career path and become a writer. I was quite offended, as it had been my lifelong goal to become a physician, like my father. But his words stuck in my head, and I have since evolved into a hybrid of the two.

When I was fresh out of residency in my full-time traditional family practice, I instinctively knew that people needed more than the communication that occurred at the office visit itself. I began to create a library of information—one-page memos on a variety of conditions that I could give the patient to take home to read. It was later that I became familiar with research that backs up the notion that people only retain a fraction of the information received during a medical visit, with a percentage of *that* understood incorrectly.

Later, after I'd become managing editor of a professional newswire for healthcare professionals, I began to realize again how fallible medicine can be, and how good health so often lies squarely within our control. If I could just pull back the curtain and show readers how small actions and lifestyle tweaks could overhaul their health and require less intervention from the healthcare system, people would be empowered to take action.

My wish for you: never be a patient. Once you see yourself as a patient—in other words, someone who is sick—that identity can take over your life. Instead, be a seeker of health. And focus on what is right in front of you. Thinking too far down the road and worrying about what may or may not come is overwhelming and can set you up for failure. There are opportunities every moment to make healthful decisions, and over time this string of beneficial choices makes a real impact.

Mindfulness—in other words, taking deliberate actions and paying more attention to your health and current surroundings—will help you get better health for less money and with less use of healthcare services.

Still, the ultimate challenge of the serenity prayer remains: how do you know the difference between the problems that the healthcare system can and can't change? Let us help you discover it for yourself, with this new way of finding better health with less expense.

To the journey,
Dr. Cindy Haines

1

Health Care: Do We Need as Much as We're Using?

*W*hat can the American healthcare system do for *you* today?

If you're sick, or injured, or dying, you're in the right place for treatment options. Stretching out from sea to shining sea, you'll find a highly trained army of roughly 900,000 doctors, physician assistants, and nurse practitioners who can provide services to meet your health needs. You have access to drugs, medical devices, and surgical procedures that would have been regarded as miraculous a generation ago—or in some cases even a decade ago.

Our doctors are educated in medical schools that are the envy of the world. We can run tests that measure hundreds of chemicals and cells swirling around in your body. We can peer into your very DNA to measure which drugs should work best for you now and which diseases might strike you decades down the road. We can put you into a big machine that literally jars the protons in your body to produce crisp pictures of your internal organs.

Sound appealing? We haven't even scratched the surface on what the healthcare system can do for you. Really, what would you like? It's all waiting for you.

How about medications? We can provide drugs that make your cholesterol go down and your mood grow brighter. We can give you drugs that help you grow more hair, make less stomach acid, help you urinate more and lower your blood pressure, or relax your bladder to cut down on your trips to the bathroom. We have drugs that open up your airways so you can breathe better, drugs that make your bone density go up, and drugs that make your blood sugar fall. We even have a prescription drug that can make your eyelashes longer.

Or are you in the market for high-tech treatments? We already mentioned one machine that shows us details of your hidden tissues and organs. That's old news. If you have cancer, you can lie on a table inside a room that looks like it was taken off the space shuttle while a beam of protons zaps the tumor. Or a surgeon can use a robot to provide better control while doing delicate surgery deep within your body.

Speaking of surgery, that's where the healthcare system can *really* work wonders. Doctors can put little tubes into the arteries of your heart through a tiny incision in your leg, and you can be home the same day! This is commonplace nowadays. We can treat back pain by fusing the bones in your spine together. These surgeries are also common. We can reroute your digestive system so you lose hundreds of pounds. We can connect you to a machine that will do the work of your kidneys. Or we can give you a *new* kidney. Or heart. Or lung. Or liver. Or even a new hand or face! Check back next year and your tireless healthcare industry will be doing even cooler stuff.

These indeed are wonderful times. Every day, American researchers are learning the secrets and solving the puzzles that have been mystifying humankind for thousands of years. When it comes to controlling disease and postponing death, American doctors now have the tools and knowledge that humans struggled for centuries to attain.

And as the scientists make new discoveries, our society wants to enjoy their benefits. During the past few decades, a steadily growing number of issues that bother us have become regarded as medical problems. Experts call this "medicalization." When people encounter an uncomfortable, embarrassing, or simply unwanted physical or mental symptom, they increasingly look to doctors to solve it, whether it's dry eyes or restless legs, hyperactivity, menopause, erectile dysfunction, or PMS. If an aspect of the human experience could *possibly* result in harm to our health, such as childbirth, our society often puts it into the hands of medical experts. That's not to say that these problems aren't worthy of treatment or medical supervision, but it does serve as a reminder of how deeply rooted health care has become in our lives.

But medicalization comes at a high cost. A 2010 study from the journal *Social Science & Medicine* estimated that twelve medicalized conditions—including male-pattern baldness, menopause, normal pregnancy and delivery, erectile dysfunction, and sleep disorders—ran up $77.1 billion in direct healthcare costs in 2005.

Medical language has escaped the halls of hospitals and medical schools and has become commonplace in homes. Our game shows and sitcoms now advertise drugs directly to consumers, bypassing the medical professionals who would have been the only audience able to understand these long words not so long ago. People thumb through health magazines in supermarket checkout lines, and they surf the Web for hours learning about diseases.

As a family physician, I am just one tiny cog in the massive healthcare industry. But in my office I get to witness firsthand the amazing ability of our medical system each and every day. Here on the front lines, I get to be part of the solution that Americans have come to expect for so many of their problems. It's a great job, and I'm grateful that I get to direct the power of our healthcare resources toward fixing my patients' illnesses.

I know that I can treat most of their problems using the knowledge and equipment I have in my own office. At other times, I can help my patients by directing them to my colleagues who specialize in brain cancer, diseased heart valves, or other specific illnesses.

In my office, I see how individual patients use health care in their daily lives. But that's just one of my jobs. My other main gig gives me a big-picture sense of how large and powerful our healthcare system has become . . . and the dark clouds that are looming on the horizon. But it also allows me to gain perspective on what we—as healthcare providers and healthcare recipients alike—can do about it. I manage the daily flow of a medical-information news service that summarizes thousands of medical studies every year for physicians and other healthcare professionals. This allows our increasingly time-crunched healthcare providers to easily stay up-to-date on new developments in their field. As a result, a constant flow of cutting-edge medical information scrolls across my computer screen every day.

This new research reminds me and my fellow doctors that our healthcare system can accomplish results that some people call miraculous. It *does* often live up to the image that you'd expect from those billboards you see along the highway, touting the latest world-class advances at your local hospital. The breadth and depth of medical knowledge in the United States should be a source of pride.

But the articles in these leading medical journals also tell another story these days. Yes, Americans have an insatiable appetite for medical care, and the healthcare system is more than willing to satisfy the public's demand—when they can pay for it.

But for how much longer can we afford this abundance of health care? As it is now, we often can't. Or we scramble to deliver this care, then find out it wasn't worth our while in the first place.

I'm frequently reading new studies that find shortcomings in drugs and surgeries that have become standard treatments. As it turns out, sometimes these don't work as well as we've been led to believe. Sometimes they don't work well at all.

In some cases, we'd be healthier, wealthier, and wiser if we said no to commonly used treatments.

In addition, millions of Americans are getting more obese and more sedentary, and experts are finding that people are setting themselves up for chronic illnesses that simply cannot be fixed in the doctor's office. Fewer and fewer people have insurance that adequately covers their medical needs. Individuals, businesses, state governments, and America itself are all buckling under the cost of all this health care. Editorials in medical journals are sounding the alarm that the healthcare system—along with the public's expectations of it—is long overdue for an overhaul.

The other common thread I see woven into this stream of news, day after day, is how most of our health afflictions, wants, and needs really require something far simpler than what health care typically delivers.

As the old saying goes, an ounce of prevention is worth a pound of cure, and this is never truer than in the case of good health. Preventing problems in the first place is ideal. But it's also true that the power lies largely within you to solve any problem not circumvented by prevention. In many cases, taking the road less traveled—or simply taking less action—might be in your best interest, and the best interest of your financial health, as well.

This notion is corroborated daily in the streams of information coming from the best and brightest minds in the healthcare industry. This kind of information is powerful and provides just the kind of fuel that can help people start to make some positive change.

In short, the fantasy that our doctors and hospitals can solve all of our problems is quickly coming to an end. The alarm is ringing, and all of us, patients and doctors alike, need to hear the wake-up call.

Sure, if you have great insurance and plenty of resources, you can still snap your fingers and have the high-tech imaging and the titanium hip replacement and the robotic surgery and the carefully aimed beams of protons. If you're still able to get any healthcare services you desire, you should count yourself among the lucky few. For now. Maybe you don't need to be concerned about saving money on your health care yet. But you probably will someday.

In today's economy, cutting-edge treatments—and even more routine medical care—are growing out of reach for working-class and even more affluent Americans. And the costs are only going to increase.

In a 2010 paper from Harvard Business School, which detailed data from 6,485 people in the United States, Canada, and several European countries, 26.5 percent of Americans said they'd cut back on routine medical care since the economic crisis. By comparison, only 5.6 to 12 percent of participants in other countries had done so. This isn't a good development. Though in many cases using less and less-expensive health care ultimately and ironically leads to better health results—as we'll say many times in the following pages—avoiding *necessary* care can actually lead to more expensive health problems further down the road.

Nowadays, when it comes to your health care, the question is no longer "What can the American healthcare system do for you today?"

It's becoming "What *can* the American healthcare system do for you today?"

Health Care: More of the Bill Is Going to You

Health care is taking an increasingly large bite out of our wallets—whether we're talking about government health agencies, employers, or individuals. Health spending reached $2.5 trillion in 2009. That's more than $8,000 for every man, woman, and child in America. Some people used far less, and many people used far more.

By 2019, which is not very far away, health spending is expected to climb to a whopping $4.5 trillion a year. Health spending already accounts for more than 17 percent of our country's gross domestic product (which, simply put, is the value of all the goods and services produced in our country during a year).

As anyone who has turned on a television or read a newspaper in recent years knows, our country's political leaders and health policy experts are wondering how we're going to pay for this, as a nation and as individuals. The tussle over health reform spilled out of Congress into town halls and talk-radio shows around the country, and listeners became familiar with some very scary numbers.

Not only are we using a great deal of expensive health services, we have an enormous number of baby boomers who will be needing more health care in coming years. The number of Americans ages sixty-five and older are expected to jump from 40.2 million in 2010 to 54.6 million in 2020. Older people spend much more on health care each year than younger adults; in 2002, according to the Agency for Healthcare Research and Quality, healthcare expenses were $11,089 annually for seniors and $3,352 annually for working-age people. A question that we should be asking ourselves is who is going to be paying for this ever-increasing healthcare bill?

The government?

It will indeed be asked to shoulder a huge chunk of the burden. Public payers—in other words, government programs (that is, taxpayers)—are expected to pay for more than half of the health care purchased in this country by 2012, according to a paper published in the journal *Health Affairs* in 2010.

But average citizens shouldn't expect the government to swoop in and start paying for all of their medical expenses. The great healthcare debates of 2009 and 2010 taught us that we Americans and our leaders are deeply divided over the role that government should play in paying for our health care.

Even with the changes that health reform brought in early 2010—which indeed provided some benefits for the public—it's a safe bet that paying for medical care is something you'll have to be concerned about for the indefinite future.

Health Reform Helpful,
But Won't Solve All Your Problems

 The health reforms enacted in 2010 provided some benefits that should help protect consumers' financial peace of mind. But even with these reforms, it's still in your best interest to look carefully at how you're using the healthcare system and find ways to make more cost-effective choices. While the new changes may offer some protection against catastrophic healthcare expenses and make it easier for you to afford health insurance, you can still be left with sizable out-of-pocket costs. And some of these protections won't start for several more years.

Here's a timetable of some significant changes we've already seen, or are expecting to see, in coming years from health reform:

2010 . . . Insurance companies can no longer deny payment when you get sick based on errors or mistakes on your application.

2010 . . . Medicare beneficiaries who hit the so-called "donut hole"—a section of expenses for prescription drugs they have to pay each year—get $250.

2010 . . . Adults younger than twenty-six can generally stay on their parents' insurance if they don't have available health coverage through their workplace.

2010 . . . Health insurance companies can't put a lifetime "cap" on certain benefits.

2010 . . . New plans must cover certain preventive services with no copays, and these services are exempt from deductibles.

2011 . . . Medicare beneficiaries will get a 50-percent discount on certain prescription drugs when they're
in the donut hole.

2011 . . . Medicare beneficiaries will get certain preventive
health services for free.

2014 . . . Small businesses will have access to tax credits
for up to 50 percent of employers' contribution to
employees' health insurance. These credits started
in 2010, for up to 35 percent.

2014 . . . Insurers will be barred from denying coverage due
to a preexisting condition. This applied to children
starting in 2010.

2014 . . . State-based insurance exchanges are set to begin.
These exchanges—along with tax credits—are
intended to help people find affordable insurance.
Tax credits are slated to be available for individuals making up to $43,000, or families of four who
make up to $88,000 who can't get other afford-
able coverage.

2014 . . . Most people who can afford it will be required to
have health insurance coverage or pay a fee.

2014 . . . Medicaid will be expanded significantly to cover
more low-income people.

Even if you have Medicare—which many people regard as
the nicest birthday present they can receive on their sixty-fifth
birthday—the amount you still have to pay can be shocking.
A 2008 report from the Employee Benefit Research Institute

estimated the amount of money that retirees will need in order to cover premiums and out-of-pocket expenses for the rest of their lives. This sum varied widely based on many factors, including your gender and the number of prescriptions you'll use. But you could be looking at spending $100,000 or even much, much more on health care during your retirement. How had you planned to enjoy your retirement? Because you could be spending a *big* chunk of your savings and retirement income on health care, even with Medicare.

Or will your insurance provider protect you from rising health-care costs? Don't bet on it anytime soon. In the first half of 2009, a survey from the Centers for Disease Control and Prevention found that 58 million Americans had been uninsured for at least part of the previous year. About 32 million had been uninsured for *more* than a year.

These days, if you lose your job—a scenario that has become all too common for Americans—you can lose your access to affordable coverage. Even if you do keep your job, your employer may no longer be able to afford to offer health insurance in the coming years. According to a 2009 story in the *Wall Street Journal,* the number of small businesses offering health insurance dropped steeply from the early 1990s—and nearly 20 percent of all companies in a survey referred to in the story reportedly planned to stop offering healthcare benefits in the next few years.

In addition, a type of insurance that's becoming more common shifts more of the cost burden to you. Known as consumer-directed health plans (CDHPs), these often combine high-deductible insurance with a health savings account. The idea here is that the insurer steps in for catastrophic injuries and illnesses, but leaves you covering the cost of more day-to-day problems. You (or your employer) can put money into your health savings account to pay for these needs on a pre-tax basis. But that's just one form of CDHP; others are becoming available as the days pass.

In 2008, according to a study in the journal *Health Affairs*, 8 percent of covered workers—about 5.5 million people—were enrolled in one of these plans, which was an increase over the 5 percent enrolled in 2007.

Insurance may become more affordable and easier to keep for Americans in a few years due to changes implemented by the recent healthcare reform. But many questions remain about how the new insurance availability will work . . . and, again, many of the changes are still years away.

However, even having insurance may not keep health costs from devastating your life. One study in the *American Journal of Medicine* found that illnesses and medical bills contributed to nearly two-thirds of bankruptcies in 2007. The majority of these people—75 percent, to be exact—had health insurance that didn't protect them from bankruptcy. Most were college-educated, owned their own homes, and had jobs that put them in the middle class.

This news can seem depressing, especially if you've not had a raise lately, you've become unemployed, you've seen your 401(k) wither, or your home is worth less than you owe on it—in other words, if you've faced the typical American's economic challenges in the past few years.

But here's some good news: Yes, rising healthcare costs are a challenge to most Americans, and America as a whole. But these costs also give us an opportunity to see our health care in a whole new light. We're getting a wake-up call that could actually *make us healthier*.

After all, what if you had a generous landlord who paid the heating bill for your home? Many people's natural instinct would be to turn up the heat to 80 degrees during the winter and bask in tropical luxury in their T-shirt and shorts. It's wasteful, yes, but if someone else is paying for it, why not enjoy it?

For many people, this has also been the case with health coverage. In years past, if you had good insurance through an employer, you might have to pay $20 to see the doctor, and a few dollars for prescriptions, and a manageable chunk if you needed to go to the hospital. But you might not have seen the *big* costs that were being paid on your behalf behind the scenes. As a result, perhaps you went to the doctor for trips that weren't really necessary. Perhaps you prodded the doctor for the latest, more expensive drug, or for a high-tech scan. Maybe you didn't carefully examine bills from the hospital after a stay. At the same time, maybe you didn't make a yearly trip to the doctor for an annual, preventive checkup that could have caught a big problem sooner. Quite possibly—as is the case for many Americans—you weren't especially concerned about your health until a problem popped up.

If this sounds like you, you're in good company. As you'll see later in this book, even doctors and hospital systems generate a lot of waste just for the sake of convenience. Test results often get lost in the incredibly complex shuffle of our healthcare system, and it can be easier to rerun blood tests and imaging scans rather than track down ones that you already had done. Unless you step up and prod your doctor to work more cost-efficiently, she may not do so.

But our hypothetical landlord isn't going to pay a huge heating bill forever. If the enormous charge became your responsibility one January, you'd likely turn down the heat to 68 degrees in a hurry. You'd put on slippers and a sweater, maybe buy an electric blanket, and your life would go on just fine. It would be different, but you'd stay warm.

The same thing appears likely to happen with health care in this country. Odds are good that one way or another, you're going to shoulder a bigger chunk of your healthcare costs. And you're probably going to want to do things differently. For example, if you have one of these high-deductible health plans, your habits may have already changed. If each year you're paying the first $1,000 or $2,000 of medical expenses that you incur, you probably care a lot more about using health services more carefully and getting a good value for the money you spend.

As you'll see in the next section, a vast fortune is wasted in our healthcare system every year. And the way Americans consume medical services is much different from the way people use their healthcare systems in other developed countries. But many Americans have confused being healthy with using health care, much in the way that someone could think being warm requires heat from the furnace. These are misconceptions we've developed.

As Eric and I were watching and discussing healthcare reform while it slowly unfolded, we read about possible solutions that the big players in health care should consider. The government should do this, insurers should do that, hospitals should do another thing differently, and doctors should shift their focus.

But we read surprisingly little about what *consumers* should do. A glance through the headlines might lead you to believe that regular people are at the mercy of these big players who have the final say on how much health care you need and how much you'll pay for it. And that's simply not true. You have a lot more power to determine how much you'll be paying for your health care than anyone has probably told you. Instead of being a passive participant in your health care, you can direct your interactions with the healthcare industry to help keep your annual costs down.

The truth is that we can often stay healthy without spending a lot of money—either our own or our nation's. A lot of the health-care costs we generate are simply unnecessary.

You can save your money while you save your health. After all, other countries are managing to do it. Why shouldn't we?

When It Comes to Health Expenses,
Our Normal Is Anything But

What else could we buy with that $2.5 trillion we spent on health care in 2009? Let's see . . . Americans seem to like the Ford Fusion car. At about $24,000, we could buy 104 million of these, which is enough to give one to most of the households in America.

Or how about one of those big white wind turbines you see popping up across the country, generating environmentally friendly electricity? At about $3.5 million apiece, we could buy 714,000 of those.

The point is, there are many things that Americans—and America itself—could be buying with our hard-earned money besides health care. So we need to make sure that we're getting a good value for the money we're shelling out.

And it doesn't appear that we are.

For all this money that our medical system is spending to treat our illnesses, Americans are not particularly healthy. We can expect to die earlier than people in Spain, Finland, Israel, New Zealand, and a host of tiny island nations. Our infant mortality rate—another sign of a society's health—is higher than the rate seen in much less-prosperous nations, including Cuba, the Czech Republic, and Iceland.

Spending more money on our health doesn't guarantee that we'll be healthier. Research has suggested that areas that spend less on health care actually have a better quality of care and better health outcomes. And people who live in areas that have had more growth in healthcare spending aren't living any longer.

That doesn't mean that our healthcare system deserves all the blame. Other factors affect the health of a population, including the way people eat and how physically active they stay from day to day. Americans on the whole have a lot of unhealthy habits, including weighing too much, eating too poorly, and not exercising enough.

Another unhealthy habit is thinking that a trip to the hospital or doctor's office can solve the effects of years of these unwise lifestyle choices.

A whopping one-third of Americans in one survey felt that "modern medicine can cure almost any illness" for those who have access, according to data published in a 2001 issue of *Health Affairs*. In Germany—the land of BMWs and, well, German engineering—only 11 percent felt this way.

We have nearly three times more MRI scanners compared to the average in many other developed nations. We have 45 percent more surgeries to reopen our coronary arteries than Norway, which has the next highest number. We spent 77 percent more on drugs per person than Japan did in 2005, noted the authors of a 2008 *Journal of the American Medical Association* commentary.

"Many people judge quality health care by *more*. If you sprain your knee now, and you can get your MRI by supper, that's quality health care," says Terry McGeeney, M.D., M.B.A. He's the president and CEO of TransforMED, a subsidiary of the American Academy of Family Physicians. His organization is working toward a number of goals to make patients better-informed users of health services who understand that less (and less-expensive) care can be the better choice.

But our fondness for high-tech treatments still doesn't explain where all that money is going. Much of our national health bill is simply wasted. The U.S. healthcare system wastes about $700 billion annually, according to a 2009 paper from Thomson Reuters. In the paper, *waste* was defined as "Healthcare spending that can be eliminated without reducing the quality of care." The authors found that of this staggering sum:

- Up to $325 billion in annual waste was on the unwarranted use of products and services. This includes antibiotics that can't possibly treat a viral infection, use of brand-name drugs when a generic drug is available, and lab tests that doctors do simply to cover themselves from a patient who might sue if they miss a problem (we'll help you trim these down in Chapter 3).
- Medical errors and provider inefficiency may run up $100 billion of needless spending. Again, you can do things to protect yourself from medical mistakes.
- Avoidable care accounted for up to $50 billion. This includes hospitalizations for conditions such as diabetes that could have been treated more effectively and more cost-efficiently earlier. You can certainly cut down on your share of this waste.

Lack of coordination between healthcare providers accounts for up to $50 billion. For example, records that don't make the trip from your specialist to your family practice doctor —or a new doctor you've begun seeing—could lead to repeated tests. Can you do something about this? Yes.

In essence, according to this report, about 64 percent of this annual $700 billion waste occurs for reasons that you can do something about. (The authors weren't even including a $200 billion annual cost of treating diseases that are preventable with behavior changes.) If we could eliminate all this waste, it would add up to about $1,469 for each man, woman, and child in America. If you have a family of four, that's nearly $6,000.

Think about this: If you bought a new car that was missing $6,000 worth of parts, you'd do something about it, wouldn't you? If you spent $6,000 on cable television each year and found out you weren't getting all the channels you were paying for, you'd be making a call to customer service, wouldn't you? If you found out that you were spending *thousands* of dollars on any other goods or services in your life that you didn't really need or weren't receiving, you'd be hopping mad, wouldn't you? You might pick up the phone and tell a representative that you wanted a solution to this problem. We're ready to see everyday Americans start helping solve the healthcare crisis in this country.

We're ready for our national conversation to discuss what *consumers* can do differently. What if all Americans saw health care as a service they should only purchase *when really necessary*? What if they demanded greater transparency in knowing how much health care costs so they could shop around and look for better deals? What if they started taking a more active role in determining which healthcare services offered the best chance of effectiveness? What if they started seeing their lifestyle choices in terms of how costly they might be for their health?

What would happen if everyone across the country opened their windows and declared: My health care costs too much, and *I'm* going to do something about it! How much money could this preserve for our government to apply to our nation's other needs? How much money could small companies save on rising insurance premiums, which they might use to strengthen their businesses or even, knock on wood, to give their employees raises or hire more employees? How much more money could families keep in their bank accounts to help see them through a rainy day?

As we've already discussed, more and more of the burden of paying for health care is being shifted to the average consumer. It's time for you to see needless healthcare expense as money that's *your* responsibility to protect.

Now, will you see an extra $1,500 per family member in your bank account at the end of the year by reading this book? That's impossible to say. Many factors will affect how much you can save on health care, depending on your type of insurance and what health problems you already have. Plus, it's hard to tally the money you *didn't* have to spend on medical care because the need for it never arose or you realized that the services weren't necessary.

But the first time you and your doctor decide you don't need a computed tomography (CT) scan that would have cost more than $1,000, think about how you'd rather spend that money you're saving. When you get a second opinion that finds you don't need a procedure to open up your coronary arteries, add that to your savings tally, too. When you enlist a billing advocate to challenge questionable charges on the bill that you incurred from a hospital trip, add those savings to the list. Making the lifestyle changes we suggest in Chapters 4 and 5 adds up, too. These are real-time savings you can start enjoying today.

This should come as welcome news to many Americans who are growing ever more concerned about the effect that high health costs are having on their families. In a survey conducted in March 2010 by Harris Interactive and HealthDay, 44 percent of adults said that they were extremely worried or very worried about paying for rising healthcare or health insurance costs.

Big savings are waiting for you, and it's time to start trimming the healthcare waste from your household budget. But the benefits don't stop there. Taking a more cost-conscious view of your health could help you reduce your yearly sick days away from work. It may help you avoid early disability, which could devastate your household finances. It may even keep you alive and provide for your family longer.

This book will give you the tools to do these things. Here's a big pair of cost-trimming scissors. Ask your doctor to grab

the other handle so you can start cutting your costs together—
because getting your doctor on your side is the first step.

The New Prescription for Finding Better,
More Affordable Health Care

The standard-issue doctor of the 1950s would be shocked by
today's patients, and vice versa. The typical physician was a white
man who was more educated than many of his patients, particularly about medical issues. He was one of the most respected
professionals in his community. His patients went in for answers
that they couldn't find anywhere else (remember—no Internet or
health channels on cable TV). The doctor told them what to do,
and they didn't question the advice. The doctor held the treatments, and the relationship was not one of equals.

And that's how it usually went.

The doctor-patient relationship of recent years has often
looked like this: The patient has already diagnosed herself based
on symptom charts that she found online. Or he's been up into
the wee hours for nights on end reading postings on online bulletin boards devoted to a condition he has.

Patients come in with information on drugs they've seen
advertised on TV. They already have an idea of what treatments
they think they need. They already know which specialist they
should *really* see if this family practice doc would just hurry
up already and write out a referral. They're taking a variety of
herbs and supplements and using all kinds of other alternative
or complementary therapies.

They're the ones often in charge now, not the doctor. It's great that patients are more involved in their medical decisions. In fact, that's crucial if they're going to get better health care for less money. However, this responsibility requires individuals to be well informed in order to make the best decisions. And often they aren't.

"If the new model is that the patients are going to be consumers, they have to be educated in order to make right decisions. We've got this really weird situation where they aren't educated or engaged. And so they think more expensive is better. You just assume the more expensive car is better than the cheaper car, and I want the more expensive car because I'm not paying anyway, whether it's a drug or other treatment," Dr. McGeeney says.

But the authors of this book think a *new* picture is going to define the way patients interact with the healthcare field. It's going to start soon—if it hasn't already. Some things will remain the same. Yes, the doctor still has good insight into your medical problems, just like in the 1950s. Yes, people are still going to be learning more about their health on their own, and coming up with ideas that they want to try based on their own research. But the new common theme running through health care will be:

- Have the doctor and I agreed on this decision together?
- Is my healthcare provider being my best advocate?
- Is this healthcare service or product really necessary?
- And if so, am I getting it for the best price?

- If not, what can I do to bring these costs down?
- Or better yet, what steps can I take to not get sick in the first place?

National medical experts will be asking many of these questions in coming years as they compare one treatment against another to see which one works better. These questions will certainly arise when you sit on an exam table in your doctor's office or prepare to go to the hospital. We suspect you'll even think more about your healthcare costs as you're going about your daily life: Which foods at the supermarket are more likely to lead to more health costs down the road? In ten years, how much will this pack of cigarettes wind up costing me?

These questions are long overdue.

After all, people these days seek out financial advisors to make sure they're taking the smart steps toward saving for retirement. Consumer-finance gurus have popular cable TV and radio shows and go on national tours, rallying crowds to live more sensibly within their means.

Given that a major proportion of our healthcare dollars are wasted, leaving people both sicker and poorer than they should be in many cases, it's shocking that no one is giving consumers the tools to stay healthier for less money. The mission statement for the *New Prescription* is: You can stay healthier for less money. Essentially this requires just four straightforward steps, and none of them are especially hard to do. Here they are:

Step #1: Work with your primary healthcare provider. You simply must develop a trusting relationship with a primary care provider who clicks with you, then you must be an active participant in your care. A huge amount of money is wasted by doctors and patients who don't understand and trust each other. Even more is wasted when patients hand over all the responsibility for their care to a doctor who's probably already overwhelmed. This is the most important step.

Step #2: Take charge of your health. It's time to realize that better health *isn't something that the doctor gives you in a pill bottle*. Being healthy is something you should give yourself, with some occasional assistance from your doctor. Having stents placed into your coronary arteries isn't a miraculous cure for chest pain. It's really a second-rate option compared to living a life that would allow you to not need such an expensive medical solution.

In addition, avoid seeing yourself as a *patient*. That implies that you're a passive participant in the healthcare system, with doctors, nurses, and hospitals bestowing health upon you. Sometimes when you start feeling like a patient, it can be hard to stop. Instead, see yourself as a person who's seeking good health—a health seeker. This healthy life may be the result of help from your doctor, but it can also be due to changes you've made on your own initiative.

Step #3: Relax about some things, but be proactive about others. We've gone from treating diseases late in the game to treating them at earlier and earlier stages. But as we're learning in some cases, looking for disease in its earliest stages can lead to unnecessary tests and treatments that are costly in terms of money and well-being. In some cases, you may be better off not looking for a problem until you have good reason to do so.

And when a symptom crops up, it may be okay to just watch it awhile to see what happens, before you have your doctor start running up your bill to treat it. We'll tell you more about the magic phrase "watchful waiting," and how it can help keep your money in your pocket—and help you avoid health care that could harm you.

However, when a problem arises that could snowball and be harder to treat later, act without delay. You don't want to end up in an emergency room on a Saturday night, racking up steep bills for a problem that could have been treated far more cheaply in your doctor's office the previous Wednesday. And you don't want to let a chronic illness cause severe damage that could have been avoided with inexpensive treatments. Nor do you want to avoid routine checkups and preventive treatments that can help keep you healthy.

In short, when it comes to your health, direct your time, energy, and money to problems only as necessary. As you'll learn in the next chapter, the best person to help you marshal your resources where they're needed is your primary care provider.

Step #4: Be a smart shopper. Buying healthcare goods and services isn't like walking down the aisles of your supermarket. It's hard to compare prices like you would by holding two boxes of cereal side-by-side. Finding out how much your local hospital would charge for a surgery compared to a hospital in a nearby community can be tough, since the information is often hard to find.

But that's changing. More people are realizing that when they schedule a surgery or visit their doctor, *they're buying goods and services*, just as if they were taking their car to the shop. As more people want to cut their health costs by comparison shopping, more hospitals and doctors who want their business will give them the information they need. We'll teach you how to find and use tools that make you a better healthcare shopper, and we'll show you how to enlist money-saving professionals to offer even more assistance.

Your New Prescription:

✓ Start seeing your health as something you help control through your everyday choices, as opposed to something a doctor provides for you.

✓ Give some thought to how much responsibility you're taking for your health. Are you doing all you can to stay well-informed about your health problems and the medications or other treatments you're using for them? Are you coming to doctor appointments ready and willing to help make decisions about your health? If not, start thinking about what you can do to become a more-informed patient.

✓ Identify your healthcare expenses and start thinking about possible ways you and your doctor may be able to reduce your need for healthcare goods and services. Could you make changes in your life that would reduce the need for medications? Conversely, do you have a chronic condition that isn't well controlled and requires expensive medical attention due to flare-ups or complications? Bringing it under better control could save you money.

2

Your Primary Care Provider and You: The Team Approach to Better, More Affordable Health Care

A *s policy makers wrestled with* fixing the problems of health care in recent years, one solution that many experts suggested was to give a more prominent role to primary care providers.

Similarly, as part of your new goal to get more effective health care at a more affordable cost, *you* must give a primary care provider a central role in your health.

Primary care physicians, by definition, include family medicine doctors, internal medicine specialists, obstetrician-gynecologists, and general pediatricians. While we'll often say "primary care physician" in this book, nurse practitioners and physician assistants are becoming more common sources of primary care, too.

Compared to many other developed countries, America has a higher ratio of specialists to primary care physicians. But placing a greater emphasis on primary care and putting one of these doctors in charge of your health care has the potential to benefit you and your health, *and* lower your healthcare costs in many ways.

Of course, I have a special interest in this, being a family medicine physician, but the research supports this idea, too. A 2009 study from the journal *Health Affairs,* looking at patients in the Medicare system, found that across the United States, when more doctors in a particular area were primary care physicians, spending per individual was lower. Another study, this one from the *American Journal of Medicine*, found that having a greater proportion of doctors in a specific area who focused on primary care was associated with less healthcare use. In fact, according to the authors, in an average-sized metropolitan area, each 1 percent increase in the proportion of primary care physicians was associated with 503 fewer hospital admissions, 2,968 fewer emergency room visits, and 512 fewer surgeries.

The association between primary care providers and lower health costs isn't the only potential benefit from having a doctor to call your own. As the authors of the second study noted, one national survey found that adults with a primary care physician had lower healthcare expenses *and* a lower risk of death. Primary care has also been linked to lower death rates from cancer and heart disease, longer life expectancy, and better overall health. Care from primary care physicians has also been linked to greater patient satisfaction and well-being.

When you think of a primary care physician, what comes to mind? A caring professional with a familiar face and office staff who have known you for years and have the skills to cover a wide range of problems? Someone who can handle your bread-and-butter needs, but doesn't have the skills or training that a specialist can offer to care for a "real" problem? Perhaps someone whose only *really* important purpose is to refer you to one of those specialists?

A study in the *Journal of General Internal Medicine* from 2000 found that patients seemed to hold conflicting sentiments about their primary care doctor. More than 60 percent of the people surveyed said they preferred to have one doctor, and a similar number preferred to get care from their usual doctor for a variety of new conditions. Almost all thought their regular doctor could handle their usual medical problems. However, 84 percent thought they should be able to get medical care from any type of doctor without a referral. And a majority thought specialists could better take care of their allergies and do a better job of prescribing medications for depression and back pain.

Specialists *should* be an important component of your overall health care—but only when they're truly needed. And I venture to say most specialists would agree. Your primary care provider is well qualified to serve as your first line of defense against illness. And if you do develop a problem that requires specialty care, your primary care provider can help you utilize those specialists more effectively and cost-efficiently. It also deserves mentioning that most specialists are overwhelmed as it is. Many specialists in my midwestern city have waiting times as long as several months. Trimming the burden of unneeded visits would help those who truly need these specialty services get what they need in a more timely, efficient, and cost-effective manner.

One of the efforts to make medicine more efficient that is gaining attention on the national scene is the so-called "patient-centered medical home," or PCMH. According to the Patient-Centered Primary Care Collaborative organization, the PCMH concept involves a healthcare setting in which:

- Patients have an ongoing relationship with a personal physician. This provider is the patient's first stop when a problem occurs. This provider also helps coordinate other services that the patient might need, including specialty care, home health assistance, and community-based services.
- The physician directs other providers within the medical home, such as nurse practitioners, physician assistants, and nurses.
- Providers use information technology to provide better care. This may include electronic medical records and methods for patients to communicate with the providers via e-mail and other Internet tools.
- The care puts more emphasis on preventive care and treating the whole person, rather than a particular condition.

According to Dr. McGeeney, whose organization, Transfor-MED, is involved in encouraging the spread of the PCMH concept, "Patients truly do need to choose a personal physician that they're going to have a relationship with. It's important for patients to not have a flavor of the month, or a flavor that's most convenient. You choose that personal physician at a time when you may have a minor illness, or need a physical exam, but you rely on that person when you have a crisis, you develop cancer, or you're in a car accident and decisions have to be made. You have to have that personal, trusting relationship already developed."

Remember from chapter 1 that our nation may run up billions of dollars in healthcare waste each year. Much of that waste is due to unnecessary care, preventable hospitalizations, and lack of coordination among healthcare providers. A good relationship with a primary care provider can cut down on *all* of these problems. Consider the following:

- Your primary doctor is a great resource to help you choose from the mind-boggling array of state-of-the-art tests and invasive surgeries—or suggest when you don't need to spend your time, energy, and money on them.
- As far as prevention goes, primary care doctors *love* to catch problems early before they bloom into more costly diseases.
- And if you do need to see specialists, your primary care doctor's office can work like a telephone switchboard operator, coordinating the efforts of other physicians and bringing their information to one location.

In short, a primary physician is the first step in your *New Prescription*. However, if you really want to get the best value from your provider, you're going to have to become an active participant in the relationship.

The New Prescription: Get Informed, Get Proactive

Let's say you were going to remodel your kitchen. The room has the same wallpaper and fixtures that came with the house when you bought it in 1991. And you're using the kitchen much more these days, so it needs new appliances and cabinets, a larger pantry, and an island.

Clearly, this is going to be a long, drawn-out procedure, requiring many decisions along the way. You're going to need help from a professional. One way to find one would be to flip through the yellow pages, poke your finger at a business at random . . . *hmm, AAA Kitchen Kontractors looks good* . . . and tell them "I don't care what you do or what it costs. Just come make my kitchen better."

Would you do that? Of course not. You almost certainly wouldn't get the results you wanted, and you'd probably wind up paying more than necessary, because for one thing, you'd have no cost comparisons and for another, you'd have to redo the work that didn't fit your wishes.

So, being the cost-conscious consumer you are, you'd instead probably shop around and get referrals from people you trust who'd gone through this experience before. You'd make an informed decision when choosing, based on your research and referrals. You'd talk to the contractor at great length beforehand to make sure you'd work well together, and to make sure the contractor has the skills, experience, and good judgment to deliver the results you're expecting. Then you'd work closely with this professional, giving your opinion on choices and making sure your home was easily accessible to allow him to work.

Unfortunately, many people put less work into their relationship with their doctor than they would a home contractor. But making sure that your health care is handled properly is far more important than a home-repair job. And it will require at least as much input from you. Simply handing over your problems to your doctor isn't the way to get better outcomes at a better price. And, frankly, letting your doctor do all the heavy lifting and decision making just isn't going to work anymore, in large part because just as our nation is realizing how much it needs primary care providers, they're becoming increasingly scarce, overburdened, and overworked.

Already, your primary care doctor may be seeing dozens of patients during a workday. She also may be doing paperwork, waiting on hold with insurance companies, and trying to reach a specialist on the phone to track down notes from a consultation that didn't arrive. An April 2010 article in the *New England Journal of Medicine* outlined the typical day for a doctor in a Philadelphia internal-medicine practice. The doctor would see eighteen patients daily. (Many primary care doctors reading this will recognize that this number seems low compared to their reality.) In addition to this, the doctor would also deal with twenty-four phone calls, seventeen e-mails, and twelve prescription refills (in addition to the prescriptions handled during visits or phone calls for other issues), and review twenty lab reports, eleven imaging reports, and fourteen consultation reports from specialists.

And when the workday is done, often the work continues with overnight, weekend, or even 24/7 call services, which many solo practice doctors must do. Your doctor may also be managing personnel issues with the office staff, worrying about covering the rent for the office this month while buying new computer equipment, and handling the other obligations of a businessperson. Because, right or wrong, that is exactly what this is—a business, and the doctor is doing a job. Doctors also presumably have a life complete with family, friends, and bills of their own to pay. Why does this matter to you as the patient (or seeker of health)? Because understanding the inner workings of a typical doctor's office, and understanding more about the doctor, will help you be a better-informed consumer, which should result in better health outcomes for you.

So the typical doctor's day is hectic, and there doesn't seem to be a break coming in primary care. The typical primary care doctor's life is likely to only get more hectic in the future. Over the next ten years, every state will need to increase its number of family doctors; however, our medical schools are graduating less than half of the number that will be needed, according to the American Academy of Family Physicians.

Medical students, burdened with their six-figure loans from med school, can make far more money in specialties like dermatology, radiology, pathology, or general surgery than in primary care—the lowest paying of the lot. A specialist can often get reimbursed a lot more money by doing a simple surgery or a diagnostic test than a family medicine doctor can get from an office visit. Some specialties may also be attractive to young doctors for quality-of-life issues such as regular hours and greater control over schedules—both in and out of the office—along with factors such as on-call responsibilities.

As a result, many overworked primary care doctors are cutting the time they spend in clinical practice, leaving the field for another occupation, or retiring from it altogether, perhaps earlier than they really would like. This, coupled with the too-low numbers of new recruits, means we are faced with a critical shortage of primary care providers. You may already have experienced the difficulty of needing to find a new doctor to take the place of one who has moved away. Or you've been faced with the challenge of needing to wait days, weeks, or even months to get in to see a new doctor, or even to see the doctor you've been seeing for years.

Another challenge? Your visit, once you get in, may be short. Faced with an increasing volume of people seeking care from shrinking ranks of providers, as well as financial pressures, the primary care providers who remain may be shoehorning more patient visits into their day, working harder and longer to make the same salary (or maybe less) than they did the year before.

In short, "Primary care, the backbone of the nation's health care system, is at grave risk of collapse," according to the American College of Physicians. They made this statement back in 2006, and the situation only continues to worsen.

So when your doctor steps into the exam room, your health issue is just one of many, many problems that she will need to resolve before her day is finished. Her job is to keep you healthy, but keeping you as healthy as possible *while saving you money* may involve extra attention from her. If you want her to look after your financial interest, she's going to want to know that *you're* going to put in the extra work that's necessary, too.

Handling Your End of a
Good Doctor-Patient Relationship

This may surprise you: Doctors usually appreciate when patients take an active role in their health . . . but they *don't* typically appreciate behavior that wastes their resources or puts them in a bind. They might not wag a finger in your face or scold you when you make life harder on them, but when you don't have a solid relationship with a primary care provider, it can change your treatment in subtle ways, and these changes might not be helpful to your health outcomes *or* your pocketbook.

As an example, here is a not-uncommon scenario that plays out in primary care offices all across our country: It's Friday afternoon and the office staff is getting ready to close up shop early that day . . . say 4:00. The on-call begins. In many practices, this means that one doctor takes on the responsibility for any after-hours phone calls that start coming in. About 4:30, the on-call doc gets a phone call from a patient—typically seen by one of her partners—who has been having a flare-up of a chronic respiratory problem since early in the week. Although the patient reports being extremely worried about his symptoms, he doesn't want to come to the office to be seen—since it's late on a Friday afternoon, after all. And this has been going on since Monday, so could the doctor just call in a prescription for antibiotics to his pharmacy?

Pitfalls to better and most cost-efficient care abound here. Let's break it down. Point one: if the patient doesn't really need antibiotics, they'd be a waste of time and money that day. Point two: needless antibiotics could set him up for drug resistance, which could lead to bigger problems and bigger bills for him down the road, wasting yet more time and money. Point three: the on-call doctor may go ahead and call in the antibiotic "just to be safe" or even "just to satisfy the patient," but the prescription is not a sure thing, or even always safe and cost-efficient in the *short* term. All medicine carries an inherent risk of side effects and other adverse reactions. So the patient could not only receive *no benefit* but, instead, could receive yet more problems that need to be treated (such as requiring treatment for an unanticipated allergic reaction), in turn costing him *additional* time and money.

And, perhaps most important, point four: this patient is not going to get the best, most cost-efficient care via a phone conversation from a doctor he has never met, for a problem that has been going on for days. Let's say that this is a viral infection on top of chronic asthma: although his condition may not be life-threatening that Friday afternoon, his chronic problem (asthma) could lead to serious consequences (respiratory distress or worse). The risk is most properly judged by seeing him in person.

Treating strangers over the phone isn't the kind of medicine I am comfortable with, and many of my colleagues feel the same way. In this example, if office hours have essentially ended, the patient could wind up going to the ER to be seen that Friday night or later on in the weekend. The average cost of a trip to the emergency room is more than $1,000. The average expense for an office visit with a primary care physician is more in the neighborhood of $100.

So these are four good reasons to not expect or even want treatment over the phone from a doctor you've never met. But here's a fifth reason, and it's a big one: it's a good way for a doctor to get sued. Why should this matter to you? Fear of lawsuits contributes to greater healthcare costs. It's not uncommon for doctors—even good, conscientious ones—to be sued. This is tremendously upsetting. The stress can take the joy right out of serving patients. Defending against a lawsuit is expensive and can occupy a doctor for years.

According to an American Medical Association survey conducted in 2007 and 2008, about 42 percent of doctors had a medical liability claim filed against them during their careers. Five percent had been sued in the previous year. Although most claims were dropped, dismissed, or withdrawn, it still cost more than $22,000 per case for doctors to defend themselves against these claims. The average overall cost to defend was found to be just over $40,000 but went as high as $100,000 or more for cases that were tried.

According to an article in the American Academy of Family Physicians' *Family Practice Management*, one of the most common reasons that family physicians are sued is for not diagnosing a disease or taking too long to diagnose it. As a result, your doctor may want to turn over every stone while seeking an explanation for your symptoms or devising approaches to your care.

Many physicians practice so-called "defensive medicine" as a way to cover themselves. In essence, these are services that are unlikely to help the patient—but may help protect the doctor from getting sued. A 2005 study in the *Journal of the American Medical Association* surveyed more than eight hundred doctors specializing in fields that are at high risk of lawsuits (such as orthopedic surgery and obstetrics/gynecology). The researchers found that more than 90 percent of those surveyed practiced defensive medicine. Ninety-two percent ordered tests, performed diagnostic procedures, and referred patients for consultation just to be safe. Nearly half had taken protective steps in recent years, such as avoiding patients who seemed like they might sue.

Another study from 2008 surveyed more than eight hundred Massachusetts doctors specializing in eight areas, including family medicine, internal medicine, surgery, and emergency medicine. Eighty-three percent said they practiced defensive medicine. The researchers calculated that 22 percent of X-rays, 28 percent of CT scans, 27 percent of MRI studies, 28 percent of referrals to specialists, 18 percent of lab tests, and 13 percent of hospital admissions were performed for defensive purposes or fear of liability.

As the authors point out, defensive medicine isn't just a matter of doing more tests. It can also include giving out unnecessary prescriptions for antibiotics, or performing invasive procedures to rule out a diagnosis or confirm it. The costs of defensive medicine could well exceed $100 billion each year (for those keeping score at home, that could be about $1,300 for a family of four).

"In my career, I always wore two hats," Dr. McGeeney says. "One was a practice I had in which I saw my patients, and the other was working in emergency rooms because I liked that adrenaline rush. If a patient came into my practice with a sprain, I'd say take two Advil and if it's not better in a day or two we'll get an x-ray. I trusted the patients, they trusted me, and two-thirds of the time they got better. I would *never* do that in the emergency room, and it's because that trust relationship didn't exist. Sometimes all this excess testing occurs because there isn't this personal, trusting relationship. When you go into an ER, you end up getting a gazillion tests because nobody trusts each other or knows each other."

So that's how defensive medicine can hurt your pocketbook. It can also hurt your health. We'll touch more on this later, but the radiation from an x-ray or a CT scan (which uses x-rays) does carry risk. The radiation can increase your risk of cancer by a small—but not insignificant—amount. Why expose yourself to this risk needlessly? Unnecessary antibiotics may leave you with bacteria that are resistant to antibiotics in the future, and you may need newer, more expensive alternatives to knock out infections down the road. And remember that each time you take a drug, you expose yourself to possible harm (such as the previously mentioned side effects or other adverse reactions) along with any potential benefit.

And speaking of possible harm, let's not forget the other risks of making journeys into the healthcare system needlessly. Our nation's doctors and hospitals save lives every day, but any treatment they use that has the power to help you also has the power to hurt you. As a prominent health-policy researcher pointed out in 2000 in the *Journal of the American Medical Association*, 12,000 deaths each year may be due to unnecessary surgery, another 7,000 from medication errors in hospitals, 20,000 from other hospital errors, 80,000 from infections acquired in the hospital, and more than 100,000 from adverse effects of medications not related to errors.

Our take-home message here is that your doctors may be inclined to do more tests and perform more treatments than are absolutely necessary, in part to protect themselves from a potential lawsuit. Of course, doctors do have other reasons for investigating every possible nook and cranny aside from litigation fears. They could be particularly conscientious, they could have trouble saying "no" to patients who demand these services, and they could just feel the need to do *something* for the patient sitting in their exam room.

But one of the central recommendations of our *New Prescription* approach is to use healthcare services only when they truly appear necessary. We've heard it said that the most expensive food you can buy in the supermarket is the food that you later throw away uneaten. Similarly, **the most expensive health care you can buy is the care that you didn't really need**. This may run counter to how your doctor normally does his job. If you ask an overworked doctor who's mindful of lawsuits to be sparing with testing and treatments, and to lean toward a cost-saving "wait and see" approach, he may be more willing to work with you if he's not worried that you'll sue if a health problem takes longer to diagnose or treat. And he'll be more comfortable working with you if he knows that you're shouldering your share of the responsibility for staying healthy.

In my experience, a doctor is much more likely to honor a "let's wait and see" request from patients who are:

- **Easily reachable.** Make sure your doctor has your contact information. This is so simple, yet so important in the doctor-patient relationship. How and where should the doctor reach you? Let her know if it's okay (or not okay) to leave a message, and if you get a message, call back promptly. Not being able to reach a patient makes it extremely difficult for healthcare providers to establish the kind of relationship that is needed for optimal care.
- **Reliable.** Doctors schedule follow-up appointments for many reasons, and your doctor might agree to put off a

follow-up in some cases. But if a patient cancels follow-ups that I think are important, I'm going to be more reluctant about letting down my guard with her care. I'm also going to have more difficulty providing cost-effective care to a patient who is "doctor shopping" or seeing specialists and other doctors on his own for a problem without my knowledge.

🖢 **Proactive.** Although sometimes better and more affordable care means *less* care, sometimes it requires *more* care *earlier*. I can have a much more cost-saving relationship with patients who catch problems early enough so we have time to treat them before they become more urgent. The patient in the earlier example with the weeklong concern who called on Friday *didn't* take this approach.

🖢 **Well informed.** As you'll see shortly, one reason doctors may need to do tests is to fill in gaps of knowledge—knowledge that sometimes can come directly from communication with the patient. If the patient can provide detailed information about her symptoms, her personal and family history of health problems, and previous tests, I may have much less need to run blood work or order imaging tests.

Hopefully we've established the importance of having a primary care provider whose guidance you trust. In the next chapter, let's look at how to find one of these professionals and start working as a team to improve your health as cost-effectively as possible.

Your New Prescription:

✓ If you don't already have a primary care provider, find one.
Don't settle for just *any* provider—choose one who will
welcome you as an equal partner in your health.

✓ Invest time in developing a good relationship with this
healthcare provider. Discuss with her how you want a *new*
type of interaction—one in which you're both going to
play a role in medical decisions that affect you. Talk about
how you're interested in saving money and using carefully
focused medical treatments.

✓ Be conscientious in your health quest. That means arriving
at appointments ready to talk about your symptoms, and
leaving appointments with an understanding of what you
need to do to address your problems. You may need to be
proactive in following up on test results and being available
if your doctor needs to speak to you.

✓ Remember that when it comes to medicine, more isn't
always better. Although situations arise that call for early
and aggressive treatment, in many cases it's wise to be
conservative with medical testing and treatments, and only
use what appears to be necessary.

3

Building a Better, More Cost-Effective Relationship with Your Primary Care Doctor

Primary care doctors and patients may want to meet each other badly enough that they're willing to go on a date (well, sort of) to launch the relationship. In 2009, a hospital in the Dallas–Fort Worth, Texas, area started a program that allowed potential patients to meet with OB-GYNs in five-minute sessions based on the speed-dating concept. The hospital was planning on expanding the program to also include pediatricians and other primary care providers.

According to an American Medical Association publication that covered the program, doctors were happy to spend an hour of their time just to pick up a few new patients who might later refer their friends and family members to the doctor. Patients could ask what the typical waiting times were for an appointment, and how long the visits lasted. They could also quickly learn if a doctor shared their thoughts on, say, alternative medicine or hormonal treatment during menopause. The doctors could suggest other physicians if a patient probably needed a different type of provider. And *everyone* could improve their chances of "clicking" with the other partner in their two-person relationship.

This appeared to be the only program of its kind in early 2010. I suspect that in today's climate, given the shortage of primary care doctors, most physicians should have no trouble finding more than enough patients. However, this story does illustrate that primary care providers appreciate having a good match with patients.

Research is finding that having a doctor with whom you see eye-to-eye may help keep you healthier. A study from the May 2010 *Journal of General Internal Medicine* followed 244 patients with diabetes and high blood pressure who visited eighteen primary care doctors. In patient-doctor pairs that had similar beliefs on how much control patients have over their health outcomes, patients were more likely to use their medications as directed compared to doctor-patient pairs in which the patients felt more strongly about their personal control than the doctors.

Find Your Best Doctor-Patient Fit

With a little prep work, you can help achieve a rewarding connection with a primary care doctor. Here's how:

See who's available. If you have health coverage, make sure to construct a list of providers in your area who participate in your network. A few minutes of research will show you which ones meet your basic criteria. Do you prefer someone younger and more recently out of training, or do you prefer an older, more experienced provider? Is it important to you that your doctor utilizes office technology such as electronic medical records or has approved the use of secure e-mail communication with his patients? Do you care if your provider is male or female? Do you have a particular language need?

Give some thought to the provider's location. Is it easily accessible from your workplace, home, or other place where you spend a lot of your time?

Ask around. Talk to your friends, relatives, and coworkers to see if they'd recommend their physician. Ask why they like their doctor, since their enthusiasm may be due to criteria that aren't as important to you.

Make the call. Once you find a few good candidates, call the doctor's office and ask if you can schedule a brief meet-and-greet visit, or see if an office staff member can answer some of your questions. Some doctors may offer a brief introductory consultation free of charge.

Good questions to ask include:

- Whether the doctor has a special interest in conditions that are of concern to you or your family, such as allergies, diabetes, heart disease, or menopausal issues.
- When the office is open, and if appointments are available on weekends or evenings. How long does it take to get in to see the doctor? What is the typical waiting time

when you arrive for your scheduled visit? What should you do in case of emergencies?

- Whether the doctor is willing to answer questions by phone or e-mail, and if a nurse is on staff to answer questions.

- If you'll always see the same doctor or if other physicians, nurse practitioners, and physician assistants in the practice will also be caring for you.

- Is the doctor knowledgeable and interested in helping you save money on your care? Will your doctor be willing to take a watch-and-see approach when appropriate instead of going right to testing and treatments?

- What is the doctor's approach to preventive care, such as breast exams, immunizations, pelvic exams and Pap smears for women, and prostate-specific antigen (PSA) testing for men? Has the doctor put some thought into doing screenings for disease only in the appropriate patients? Will he be willing to explain the risks of these tests before you agree to them? As you'll see in Chapter 6, these screening tests can open the door to thousands of dollars of unnecessary care, so you and your doctor should approach them with *informed* care.

- Will the doctor inform you of test results? How and when? You spent the time and money getting those tests, and your doctor should make an effort to let you know what they found. But some doctors are more prompt about this task than others. If not the doctor, then who typically calls you with test results and other office communication? As I like to—and frequently—say, "No news when it comes to medical testing is not good news. No news means they might've lost your test(s)."

While you're there, check out the "vibe" from the waiting room and the rest of the office. Is this a place where you'll feel comfortable and welcomed? Remember, ideal communication often boils down to how well you click. This factor is arguably much more important than where the doctor went to medical school or where she did her residency.

In order to obtain carefully focused medical care that only uses the services you really need, you're going to have to trust the doctor's diagnosis and recommendations. In this first meeting, do you get the sense that this is someone whose judgment you'll trust? Is she going to communicate well with you and take your requests seriously? Is she willing to share responsibility for your health with you? Is she going to be easy to reach?

Once you establish a good relationship, stick with your doctor unless you have a very good reason to move on. The name of the game in getting better care for less money is having a long-term familiarity with your doctor. Doctor-hopping costs time and money in terms of moving your records from place to place. It also increases your chances of having redundant or inconsistent care, such as needlessly repeated tests or treatments or, conversely, problems that go untreated because they fall through the cracks.

While you're at it, forge a good relationship with the other staff members at the doctor's office, such as the receptionists, nurses, and medical assistants. Many of them perform multiple roles in the office, which tends to be as busy as a beehive. Being on friendly terms with these people could help improve your odds of getting quick, effective, and cost-efficient care sometime down the road.

Be a Good Record Keeper

When you're at a doctor's office, it's not hard to notice that the healthcare field generates a lot of information. All those floor-to-ceiling file cabinets are filled with patient records. Even in the age of mass conversion to electronic medical records (EMRs), enormous amounts of paper records still stream in via fax and snail mail from specialists, testing centers, and ancillary care providers, as well as patients themselves.

Each visit to your doctor adds more paperwork: a record of your symptoms, the doctor's diagnosis and treatment strategies, the results of more tests. When you see specialists, they generate more records, too. Even if your primary doctor is linked into an EMR-keeping system, it is likely that many of the specialists and other care providers are not, or they're linked into a different (and probably incompatible) system altogether. In other words: those tests you think your doctor is getting because "they're all in the same system" may not actually be arriving.

In the old days, it may have been okay to let your doctors worry about ensuring that these reams of information got to the right place. Not anymore. Keeping your *own* personal health records is necessary these days if you want to get the best health care in our medical system. And saving money on your health care requires being a knowledgeable patient with informed opinions on the types of products and services you want. Being more knowledgeable begins with maintaining thorough information about your health.

Don't assume that your doctor will be able to obtain and track all of your health records, even if your doctor's office does have electronic record keeping. We have already mentioned how busy just one doctor and just one office can be. And we still seem to be very far away from all of the various EMRs being able to flawlessly sync their data. Thus far, the leaps made in technology have not begun to touch the age-old problem of records making it from points A to B.

Keeping a personal health record can save you money and lead to better care by:

Reducing duplicate tests. Doctors may do many tests in order to assess your health, and you may have to run back and forth between specialists to have these done. Even if these different doctors belong to the same hospital system, they may not always communicate your test results to each other very well. Doctors commonly repeat tests because they don't know you've had them already (and sometimes they repeat them because it's just easier than tracking down existing results!). By keeping a record of when you had a test and what it found, you can save yourself the hassle—and cost—of needless testing.

Tracking changes in your health. If you have a chronic condition, such as diabetes or high blood pressure, it's a great idea to keep your own log of applicable readings, such as your blood sugar or blood pressure. As we'll discuss later in the book, you can make lifestyle changes that may reduce your need for medications for these conditions. Tracking the improvements in these numbers can guide you toward gaining better control over the disease. On the other hand, if the numbers are getting *worse*, your doctor may offer more time-efficient ways to help you change your management approach and avoid costly complications.

Getting to know yourself better. As an example, keeping track of your blood pressure not only helps improve management of high blood pressure, it can also head off the diagnosis at the pass altogether. Sometimes, abnormal readings at the doctor's office can be red herrings.

A high blood pressure reading in a clinical setting could be what we call "white coat hypertension," a situation where you don't really have hypertension at all; your pressure is simply elevated in the setting of the healthcare environment. You may feel nervous about being there, or you could have been racing to make the appointment on time. Knowing what your blood pressure runs normally can point your doctor in the right direction. (It's also helpful to bring in any home blood-pressure measuring devices you use, so your healthcare team can compare the values with those obtained in the office.)

Other ways of getting to know yourself better that can lead to better health care include doing monthly breast exams for women, testicular exams for men (ages fifteen to forty), and regular skin checks (with the help of a friend or loved one who can help with the hard-to-see areas, like your back and scalp). I say that the real point of these "getting to know yourself" exercises is really just that: getting to know yourself, getting comfortable with yourself, and knowing what is normal for you. Getting to know your "normal" through regular self-exams provides the opportunity to better know when something unusual has cropped up. And this can increase the chances of finding an abnormality at an earlier stage, compared to waiting to be examined only once a year at the doctor.

Being better informed. At the very least, maintaining a personal health record keeps you involved in your health. You and your doctor should be equal partners in making your health decisions. Being well aware of your health history gives you the tools you need to make good choices as a member of this team.

In addition, if you're ever hospitalized or you develop a chronic problem that generates considerable medical charges, you may be able to save money by carefully checking your records and disputing charges with your provider or approaching your insurer if it declines payment for a service. Being familiar with your medical records could help give you a head start at these moments.

You have several options for keeping a personal health record. These include keeping your records on paper in a file folder, inputting them onto a Web-based record such as Google Health or Microsoft HealthVault, or keeping them on a computer storage device such as a flash drive. Some employers and health insurers provide services to help you maintain a personal health record. We're not going to recommend any specific type here. Just keep in mind that some types are more easily accessible (like online records), some are more portable (flash drives), and some may be easier to keep private for your eyes only (paper, kept in a locked file cabinet). If you use a service from an outside provider, be sure to find out who else has access to your information, how you can extend access to your health provider, and how you can move your information to another service in the future.

Whichever method you choose, the American Health Information Management Association (AHIMA) recommends that your personal health record include these minimum elements:

- Your personal information (name, Social Security number, date of birth)
- Emergency contact information
- The contact information for all your healthcare providers, including your dentist and specialists
- Your health insurance information
- Medications you're currently taking and their dosages
- A list of significant illnesses and procedures, along with when they occurred
- Allergies
- A record of pertinent family medical history
- Immunizations and when you received them
- Opinions from specialists
- Test results

- 🔍 Correspondence with healthcare providers
- 🔍 A living will and advanced directives (which cover issues including how much medical care you'd want if you were no longer able to speak on your own behalf)
- 🔍 Organ donation wishes

In addition, if you're tracking your blood pressure, blood sugar, weight, or other measurements that regularly change, it's wise to include these in your record, too.

To start compiling your personal health record, ask for recent records from your providers' offices each time you visit, including eye doctors and other specialists. Since your providers probably have many files regarding your care, it may be easier to gradually build your record, according to the AHIMA. And be aware that you may have to pay a fee to cover the cost of copying these records.

If you've had lab tests or imaging studies, make sure you get copies of any reports for your records. When a doctor orders these, ask when the results should be ready and when you should call to get them. It's reasonable to expect your doctor to give you this information—after all, the two of you are in a relationship of shared responsibility and respect. That being said, test results are one of those things that a doctor's office is apt to not pass along unless you give them some prodding. If you don't get the results on time, don't get upset; just make the call and ask for the information.

Nationwide, a movement is growing to shift providers' records to an electronic format that doctors can share more quickly and easily. Some doctors' offices and hospitals are further along in switching than others. As you start to build your personal health record, talk to a staffer in your doctors' offices to see if they have electronic records that they can easily copy for you to keep in your files or put on your computer.

Once you create this repository of health information, your doctor is *not* going to want to sift through the entire thing at every visit. Instead, refer to your records as needed before an appointment and jot down specific information you think will be relevant. For example, if you're going to be talking about your blood pressure, make note of any recent changes and overall trends. Also jot down basic information on any visits you made to other specialists, or on any tests you've had since your last visit. Better yet, bring those test results with you so your doctor can make a copy for her files.

Help Your Provider Make
an Accurate Diagnosis More Quickly

Between 1997 and 2005, the average length of an appointment with primary care doctors actually increased from eighteen to nearly twenty-one minutes, according to a 2009 study from the *Archives of Internal Medicine*.

That may sound like a lot of time, especially if your doctor seems more like a white-coated blur who pops in and out of your visits. However, doctors appear to be cramming more tasks into a typical visit these days. Another study, published in the *Journal of General Internal Medicine*, found that during this same period, the number of "clinical items" covered in each visit increased from 5.4 to 7.1. These items included making diagnoses, discussing medications, ordering tests, and counseling patients. My experience isn't much different. As I also have found over the years, once you factor in all the business that needs to be covered, including note taking, this isn't much time at all.

The bottom line here remains: you don't have any time to waste in the typical visit. In order to come up with a well-reasoned, cost-efficient, and effective approach to your problem, it's important that you and your doctor get the most value from this time.

Start by describing your issue as efficiently as possible. This may help your doctor make the correct diagnosis and recommend better options the first time. Getting the right diagnosis, and proceeding with the right treatment, is crucial for getting the best and most cost-effective health care. Seems pretty basic, right? Yes, it is a basic premise, but much of the waste in our healthcare system (and poor outcomes despite overall higher costs) can be directly attributed to inefficiencies from the outset. The correct diagnosis and treatment plan from the get-go can, in many cases, save you the time and expense of trying treatments that don't work, making return visits to change the approach, undergoing unnecessary testing, or needing to visit specialists. Here's how to help your doctor on this task:

Get there early. I know—doctors always seem to be running late. Why show up early just to spend more time in the waiting room? Because if we *all* showed up a little early for appointments, the doctor would be better able to stick to a timely schedule. It only takes a few patients being five minutes late to create a snowballing effect that wreaks havoc on the doctor's entire schedule for the day. By arriving a few minutes early, you'll have time to update your insurance, fill out forms, and do any other administrative business that may be required. If you have the choice, make your appointment earlier in the day or first thing after the office's lunchtime, since odds are better that your doctor won't have encountered a delay yet.

Bring written reminders. If you need help remembering the problems that are bothering you or the questions you want to ask your doctor, write them down. Sitting semiclothed in an exam room can be a little disorienting, and having a written reminder of what you wanted to discuss can help you steer the visit in the direction you need. With the time you may spend waiting for your doctor, you can get your ducks in a row by reviewing your notes on what you want to talk about that day, what you hope to accomplish, and any questions you would like to have answered.

Make your list but limit your focus. Although it may seem efficient and cost-effective to stock up seventeen health concerns for one visit to your doctor, it's not. Your doctor isn't going to have time in this brief visit to handle all of them satisfactorily. On your written reminder note, prioritize the concerns you want to discuss, and be sure to start with the top one. When the doctor comes into the room, ask how much time he will be able to spend with you. Consider letting the doctor see your list, so he can help you pick out the most pressing concerns.

If your doctor doesn't think you'll have time to cover them all, discuss making a follow-up appointment for the less time-intensive problems. Before you get annoyed at having to come back, know that you can make this work for your benefit. Trying to cram everything into one visit may well end up shortchanging the care you receive. Splitting concerns across two or more follow-up visits will not only allow more time for each, but will also allow the opportunity for you to more comprehensively review what happened at that last visit and follow up on anything left hanging.

And whatever you do, try to avoid the "doorknob drive-by," also known as the "Oh, by the way." This is the problem that just happens to pop into your head (or the one you've really come for but felt too shy, nervous, or embarrassed to bring up at the outset) after the doctor has said her good-byes and is on the way out the door. You're simply not going to get the most effective care if you bring up your problem at this point. If it's something embarrassing that you had to work up the nerve to mention, it still would have been better to discuss it sooner. (Trust me: whatever you mention, your doctor has seen or heard of something more unusual.)

Be able to describe your symptoms thoroughly. When my father (who is a family doctor, too) was in medical school, a professor once told him that "Medicine is simple: just listen to the patients and they will tell you the diagnosis *and* the treatment." In the old days, before we had million-dollar imaging devices and a myriad of lab tests, that's all doctors had—listening to the patient and doing physical exams. And, ironically, that was often enough.

Even today, high-tech diagnostic tools should only play a small role in helping your doctor diagnose a medical problem. The important variables for your doctor—comprising most of what she needs to do her job—come directly from you. No machine can measure a sensation you feel deep inside as well as you can explain it.

So, when you discuss your concern, be ready to describe it in great detail, as if you were telling a friend about a movie you saw. Is your pain sharp or dull? When did it start? What were you doing when it started? Does it come and go? Does it occur at specific times of day? Can you do anything to relieve the pain? Does anything you do make it worse? Do you have any other symptoms that might be related? If you are a reproductive-age female, do you know the date of your last menstrual period? The clock is running, so have this information ready to go.

The more detail you can provide about your symptoms when the doctor asks, the better. Many problems, from minor to serious, can cause chest pain. The better you describe it, the better your doctor can pick a smart approach. Similarly, specific descriptions such as a "spinning sensation" or "lightheadedness" versus "dizziness" all have a particular meaning to your doctor. Your doctor has many paths to choose between when seeking a diagnosis, and your words are the signposts that point him in the right direction.

Refrain from offering your own diagnosis. Any number of websites will let you enter your symptoms, then provide you with possible diagnoses. It's fine for you to research your condition before you arrive at the doctor's office, but try to refrain from starting the conversation with "I think I have X. Here's why."

Your doctor will develop a list called a "differential diagnosis" in his mind during your visit. This is the list of all the different things that could be causing the symptoms you describe. As he decides on which one seems most likely, he's going to be weighing many factors aside from your symptoms that you probably *didn't* tell the website: your age, your weight, your family history of diseases, whether you're under stress at work, and so forth. Your doctor will devote plenty of mental resources toward thinking through all the options on this list. This is the part they do best, and it's probably wise for you to contribute the information that *you* know best—which is describing your symptoms, rather than swaying the doctor in a specific direction at the outset.

Know your family history. Medical conditions can be passed from generation to generation through the genes. As a result, if other people in your family have developed a disease, you may also have the genes that put you at higher risk. In some cases, your doctor will better be able to diagnose and treat a condition if you can provide information on your family risk. Will this be useful if you have a sprained ankle? Highly unlikely. If you may have colon cancer, heart disease, diabetes, dementia, arthritis, or high blood pressure? Yes.

Try to have information available on at least two to three generations of your family; however, the more you know about closer relatives the better. This includes parents, siblings, and children (which are your first generation), aunts, uncles, and grandparents (second generation), and great-aunts, great-uncles, first cousins, and great-grandparents (third generation). For this genetic family history gathering, you're only concerned about blood relatives—not relatives by marriage (and not neighbors or family friends).

A study from the March 2010 issue of *Gastroenterology* that involved records on more than 2.3 million people found that those with a first-degree relative (parent, sibling, or child) who has had colorectal cancer are at higher risk of also getting the disease. But also having distant relatives who have had colorectal cancer can make the risk go even higher.

If your doctor has a need for family information, he'll probably only want to know who had the condition; at what age the condition started; if the relative had any other factor that may have contributed to the condition; and, if the relative is deceased, what he died of and at what age. Although it can be tempting to spend a lot of time discussing family, your primary care doctor probably just wants a brief recap here.

Don't deliberately try to "visit" by phone. Some patients may try to save themselves the cost and time of an office visit by simply calling the doctor's office after hours. You may be able to get what you want from your doctor this way, but it comes with a significant risk of misdiagnosis or mismanagement of your problem, since the doctor probably won't have access to all your information or files, can't see you in person, and may miss valuable clues. Come into the office for a face-to-face visit if possible.

Help Your Doctor Devise a Better, More Cost-Effective Diagnosis Plan

The next time you're in a crowded restaurant, take a look around you. Each person you see in the room probably has *something* going on inside that a curious doctor could find interesting enough to investigate further. You probably do, too. If money weren't an option, we could do blood tests and almost certainly find that *some* specific factor is a little too high or a little too low, or is just at the edge of normal. Does it mean that something is wrong with you? Probably not. Does it mean that something is *going* to go wrong with you? Again, probably not. Could we spend a great deal of money investigating it and giving you some kind of treatment for an issue that you didn't know you had? Of course—and that happens all the time.

In general, this book's approach for better and more cost-effective health care involves careful use of testing. And it follows this philosophy: "Treat the patient, not the lab results." Clearly, you want your doctor to use lab tests and imaging tests when they're necessary. But before you ask for general screening labs that may not be indicated, or if there is no clear reason why your doctor is recommending a test, proceed with caution. As we'll discuss in much greater detail in later chapters, tests come with risks. I'm not only talking about the immediate risk of having blood drawn or being exposed to radiation, but the risk that this information will lead to additional tests or even some kind of treatment that you don't really need. Not to mention the very real risk of the anxiety that can come when you get news that something could be amiss with your health.

How will you know if you would benefit from any given test, or if your doctor genuinely thinks she needs this information to offer necessary medical care, or if she's doing it for some other reason? Ask. If you have a trusting relationship based on shared decision making, your doctor will be happy to tell you why she thinks you do or do not need any requested or recommended test. During this discussion, consider the following questions:

How will any information that you find change my treatment? Can your doctor treat you just as well *without* this information? In many cases, your doctor can choose a reasonable course of action without additional testing. As an example, one of my close family members recently had what appeared to be a transient ischemic attack, which is also known as a mini-stroke. But be careful of the lingo: these aren't so minor. In fact, these often serve as a warning that you have a higher risk of a full-blown stroke down the road, so you want to get these checked out.

His primary doctor sent him to a neurologist, who recommended an MRI with gadolinium, which is a contrast agent that enhances the image. Despite attempts to retrieve his test results, he never did hear back from his neurologist, and he ultimately had to get them from his primary doctor. Did having this expensive test change his doctor's approach? No. Did my family member ask whether his doctor really needed this test? No. But he will from now on, because it does make a difference. Taking any action requires knowing about the pros and cons that come along with it.

What are the pros and cons of this test? X-rays and CT scans expose you to radiation and can increase your risk of cancer. In 2006, Americans received about 377 million radiologic procedures (including x-rays and 67 million CT scans), and 18 million nuclear medicine studies, which involve ingesting, inhaling, or having an injection of radioactive material. From 1950 to 2006, diagnostic radiologic exams increased nearly tenfold. Per person, the annual effective dose from medical procedures (a term used with radiation exposure) in America is among the highest in the world, and it appears to have risen 600 percent from 1980 to 2006, according to a 2009 article in the journal *Radiology*.

But even tests that don't involve radiation, like the MRI my family member had, can involve risks. He had ongoing pain in his arm where the gadolinium was injected into his hand and, in researching this as a side effect, he discovered that gadolinium is associated with kidney-related concerns in some people. Had he known this earlier, especially along with the knowledge that any results from the test would not have an impact on his care, he would not have consented to the expensive and time-consuming test. Not to mention the time and energy he spent worrying about the arm pain he wouldn't have had, and the time spent researching the test and its side effects.

It's one thing if a test brings plenty of potential benefit to weigh against its potential risks. But if it's not particularly useful for your doctor, ask if it's really worth the investment of your time, energy, and money.

Can I deal with the information? Not only is it important for the doctor to know what to do with test findings, you should also consider how you'll handle this information. When I was pregnant with my second child, I had an experience with a screening that left a big impact on how I think about medical tests. I was going to be thirty-five at the time of my child's birth, and a physician friend suggested that I have a test at around eleven weeks to check the baby for chromosomal problems, including Down syndrome (the "first trimester screen"). The idea was that I'd get reassurance much earlier as opposed to waiting for the more traditional "triple screen" blood test at around sixteen weeks. This test was relatively new at the time and has since become much more mainstream, especially for women of so-called advanced maternal age, like I was.

Another plus? This test is noninvasive, meaning no risky chorionic villus sampling (CVS) or amniocentesis. Just a simple ultrasound—we do them all the time—coupled with a blood test and bingo! . . . you can cross a worry off your list ahead of time.

So I went in and had the test at eleven weeks. After all, what harm could the screening test do? It was quick and indeed fairly noninvasive, involving just the blood sample and that ultrasound to measure tissue at the back of my baby's neck. And it would allow me to check one more thing off my list, which for a pregnant mom with a busy toddler and full-time job can grow long.

But the test neither relieved my worry nor checked something off my list. No—it added to both. The test suggested that my baby might have a problem. The words "suggested" and "might" are critically important because this is a *screening* prenatal test, not a *diagnostic* prenatal test. In other words, this test could only give a ballpark estimate of what the chances were of a certain diagnosis—in this case, the likelihood that my baby had a chromosomal abnormality, ranging anywhere from mild to severe and possibly not even compatible with life. A diagnostic test, in this scenario, would be the more invasive CVS (a first trimester test that requires a sample of part of the placenta, the chorionic villi) or amniocentesis (typically done in the second trimester via extraction of amniotic fluid). While the risk of both of these procedures is low, it is important to know that each is not risk-free. Along with the benefits of getting information on the health of the baby (and, possibly, relieving parental anxiety), come the risks, including bleeding, infection, harm to the baby, and even miscarriage.

Abnormal first trimester screens have also been associated with an increased likelihood of finding heart defects, as well as some other health issues like diaphragmatic hernia, that can be targeted more accurately for diagnosis via a detailed ultrasound later on in the pregnancy.

So the screen can give you a heads-up on issues you may need to know about for your baby's sake. Still, what I did not give enough—or perhaps more accurately, *any*—thought to prior to getting this test was the risk of getting a false positive or a false negative. A false positive means the test has identified a cause for concern that doesn't really exist. Knowing that the majority of positive first trimester screens are, in fact, falsely positive, may have influenced my decision. On the other hand, a false negative means the test *didn't* identify a disease or a risk that is *actually* present. It is just as important to acknowledge that getting word that the risk of a certain health outcome is low based on a screening test does *not* mean that you have definitively ruled it out nor, as in this scenario, does it mean that you can have a 100 percent expectation of a healthy child.

For this screening, about 85 out of every 100 babies affected by the abnormalities addressed by the test will be identified. A positive result will be given to somewhere in the neighborhood of 5 percent of all normal pregnancies. Getting this positive test result means that you have anywhere from a one in 100 to one in 300 chance of the baby actually *having* one of the abnormalities for which you're being screened, according to the American Pregnancy Association.

So now faced with this information and having made my decision that I did not want to take on the risk of additional testing, I proceeded to do what many people do in the face of medical uncertainty and feelings of powerlessness: I got online and caught a bad case of what I call "Google-itis." I combed through mountains of information on the test, and what the results could mean, and how our family would need to make adjustments to accommodate a child with additional needs—should that indeed be the outcome.

After several weeks of obsessing over these test results, one of my doctors told me that just the *worrying* could actually be harming my baby. So at twenty-one weeks, I agreed to an amniocentesis to give me the definitive diagnosis for my baby regarding what we could expect chromosomewise. This test provided the diagnosis that the first test could only estimate: There were no chromosomal issues. The other issues of potential concern (such as a heart defect) were more fully evaluated via an ultrasound around week twenty. Our son was expected to arrive 100 percent healthy (as he did). For me, the early screening exercise—and the false positive result it brought—was all for naught.

I spent two months of my pregnancy worrying for no reason —two months of *suffering*. And my doctor was right: All that worrying was certainly not good for my unborn child nor was it good for my toddler daughter or my concerned husband, not to mention the rest of our family. So what good could I have gotten from the first screening? In this particular case, for me, I realize there really wasn't any upside. Regardless of what the test found, I was going to continue my pregnancy. Any major health issue that may require intervention rapidly after birth (such as certain heart defects) could be more accurately assessed via a second trimester ultrasound (which I was going to get anyway). So the results wouldn't have changed *any* of my decisions. Yes, there is value in being able to prepare yourself for a particular outcome. But, in essence, I asked for information without considering that I might not get the news I wanted to hear. I asked for information that I did not need, which led to great distress over a potential diagnosis that never even came to be. Why did I do it? For the same reason you might consider any screening test as well: I expected to get the results I wanted to hear—that all was well and there was no need to do anything else.

So before the doctor does any kind of testing, don't just ask what he will do with the results. In other words, ask him: "Is this necessary? Will a positive result be a definitive diagnosis or will it mean more testing? What are the next steps if and when we get a positive result?" Also ask yourself: "Do I even *need* this information? Will this information change anything about my healthcare plan? If this info is not 'need to know,' can I keep calm if I get news that may not be what I want to hear?"

Help Your Doctor
Devise Cost-Effective Treatment

Once your doctor has a hunch about what may be causing your problem, he'll move on to how it should be treated. Here's a little piece of information that may surprise you: The "right" treatment for a health problem is seldom set in stone. If you get ten doctors in a room devising a course of action for a condition, you'll likely get ten approaches that are at least *slightly* different.

Does that mean that nine of the doctors are wrong? No. It just means that many times in medicine there's no one right answer. And doctors tend to use the treatments they're accustomed to providing. "An awful lot of cardiologists are going to want to do a cardiac catheterization if you're having chest pain," Dr. McGeeney says. "If you go to a back surgeon, they're going to want to operate on your back. But usually in six months, the vast majority of back pain is going to get better no matter what you do. Surgeons want to operate. But if you go to your primary care doctor, they're going to try physical therapy, medications, and that kind of thing."

As a result, you and your doctor often will have room to maneuver when you're putting together the most cost-effective approach that uses only the necessary amount of treatment. As you and your doctor develop your treatment together (remember that *shared* decision making is the name of the game), ask the following questions:

Will this problem go away on its own? A fundamental component of the *New Prescription* approach involves watchful waiting. Some experts call this "active surveillance." In essence, it means you watch a problem to see if it clears up on its own, or at least doesn't get any worse. You and your doctor aren't doing nothing; rather, you're looking before you leap into a treatment.

Whether it's watching young kids with an ear infection for a while before prescribing antibiotics, or observing a man with a prostate tumor that appears nonaggressive before proceeding to surgery, experts these days are more frequently exploring when watchful waiting may be a good idea.

Some problems are self-limiting, meaning that they'll get better by themselves whether you take a medication or not. Ask your doctor if your symptoms are likely to clear up without requiring you to buy a medication. Discuss whether your doctor can prescribe or recommend a treatment that you can use a little later if the problem doesn't look like it will go away on its own. Discuss when you should be seeing improvement, what the warning signs will look like if the problem is getting worse, and at what point you should start using the treatment. Some doctors may even give you a prescription to fill at a designated point if symptoms don't resolve—or begin to worsen—within a certain time frame.

Let's be clear that watchful waiting isn't useful for every condition. For example, doctors now may treat rheumatoid arthritis aggressively early after diagnosis, to help limit joint damage from the disease. Again, your doctor is your best ally in terms of recommending whether you truly need treatment, when early treatment is the best approach, or if you may benefit from a wait-and-see approach.

What can *I* do to make myself better? For some problems, you may be able to avoid having to take medications—or you may need less of them—just by losing weight and exercising more. Diabetes and high blood pressure are two examples. You'll save money and be healthier overall if you make good lifestyle changes instead of just taking daily pills for these problems. If you're having headaches or trouble sleeping, you may get better relief from cutting out caffeine, asking your partner to rub your shoulders, or finding solutions to a source of stress in your life than from taking a pill.

No matter what your condition, discuss what *you* need to bring to the table to maintain better health. If you can do more to stay healthy on your own for free or little cost, doctors may need to use fewer expensive approaches further down the road. The best medicine is the kind you never have to take. We're fortunate to live in an age where we have so many medications available to us, but the goal is still to use them as sparingly as possible, and if you do have to use them, only use them for a short time.

Are we understanding each other? Sometimes doctors and patients have a hard time communicating about medical problems and moving forward toward a solution. This may occur when the problem you're working on involves symptoms that are proving difficult to manage, such as some cases of chronic pain. Patients can get frustrated, feeling that the doctor isn't understanding or being helpful enough, or they get the sense that they're being brushed off. Doctors can get frustrated that the solutions they're trying don't seem to be working, or they may feel that the patient is being pushy or has unrealistic expectations. And the collaborative attitude that is so vital to this relationship can become replaced with a sense of defensiveness and impatience.

If you're facing a medical problem that's difficult to treat, try to stay patient and calm. Sometimes problems take time to solve. Sometimes there may not be a treatment that's as effective as we would all like. Sometimes doctors and patients have to work through different approaches to find one that's the most helpful.

If you and your doctor have reached an obstacle in your ability to communicate about your symptoms, try a different approach—rather than repeating attempts to get your point across that haven't worked already.

Is a less-expensive drug available? The commercials for drugs that you see on TV during popular shows, with the famous actresses and computer-generated graphics, cost a lot of money. And that cost gets passed on to you when you buy them. Hopefully you've read enough already that this bit of advice won't surprise you: don't insist that your doctor prescribe a new drug just because you saw it in an advertisement.

In some cases, a new drug may indeed be the best one for you. However, if your doctor wants to try an older drug instead, it's probably for a good reason. Perhaps he thinks it will work for you based on previous research, or he has similar patients who have done well with it in the past. Maybe he's seen too many hot new medications in the past that failed to work as advertised or wound up being harmful.

Sometimes, despite the availability of increasing numbers of newer "designer" options for a condition, the older standbys may do the job just as well—and cost a lot less. Remind your doctor that you're interested in the best *and* most cost-effective approach to your treatment. If he's choosing between several drugs that could be helpful, he may be able to prescribe one of the less-expensive options.

Be sure to ask your doctor if generic medications are available. Although the media have carried stories in the past few years questioning the safety and effectiveness of generic versions of brand-name drugs, generics are typically a sensible choice. They have the same active ingredients as their brand-name versions, and they're often available at a fraction of the cost. We'll talk about these more in Chapter 8.

And finally, ask if your doctor knows the cheapest place to obtain the medication. In recent years, some supermarkets have begun offering drugs, including antibiotics and the diabetes medication metformin, free of charge. It's a bad idea to take a drug that you don't really need just because it's free (taking needless antibiotics can lead to higher health costs further down the road), but if you truly need the drug, you can't get a better price than free.

Are over-the-counter medications or other treatments safe or helpful? You may be able to treat your problem more cheaply using an over-the-counter medication. Conversely, in some cases these may do little to make you better any faster or ease your symptoms. Your doctor can offer some insight on whether an over-the-counter drug will be helpful or just a waste of money.

And ask if nonmedication approaches may also be helpful. If you're having balance issues due to age or a medical condition, having grab bars in your bathroom can save you from a costly injury. Orthotics in your shoes may help relieve hip or back problems. Wearing special support hose may help prevent blood clots in your circulation that can trigger extremely serious (and expensive) complications. Your doctor may not think to mention these other tools unless you ask about them.

Could talking to your pharmacist help? Pharmacists may be often-overlooked professionals in your healthcare team who can save you money and improve your care—if you talk to them. Policy makers are considering ways that pharmacists can take on more responsibilities in keeping patients healthy in coming years. Get on a first-name basis with a pharmacist, and if you have a medication-related question, run it past him or her.

What Is a Physician Extender?

 In coming years, as new patients begin flooding into the primary care system, odds are good that you'll be encountering physician extenders more often. This isn't a piece of equipment that allows a doctor to reach out further, but it's a similar idea.

This is a term that encompasses healthcare providers who aren't doctors, such as nurse practitioners (NPs), and physician assistants (PAs). These professionals may have different responsibilities—and require different levels of supervision from a doctor—according to different state laws. But the services they may provide include diagnosing and treating illnesses, prescribing medications, performing diagnostic tests, and doing exams.

If your doctor's office makes use of these providers, they can also help the doctor focus on patient issues that demand a doctor's unique skill set. And as already-busy primary care offices become even busier, PAs and NPs may become crucial in your mission to get great health care at a reasonable price.

If your doctor's office asks you to meet with a PA or NP at your next visit, give them a chance instead of immediately asking for a doctor. You may be able to get in more quickly to see an extender rather than the doctor, and this provider may be able to spend more time with you. You may also be equally pleased with the results. A 2000 study published in the *Journal of the American Medical Association* of 1,300 patients who met with either a doctor or an NP found that both groups had similar satisfaction with the visit afterward and six months later, and similar health status six months later and use of health services after six months and one year.

Your New Prescription:

✓ Know your body and your symptoms. If you have a health complaint, be ready to answer any question your doctor has about it.

✓ Keep good records on your conditions and treatments.

✓ Understand the risks and benefits of any test or treatment your doctor offers. Are they really necessary? Will the results of the test affect the way your doctor handles the problem? Can the treatment be postponed for a while to see if your symptoms will go away on their own? Can you take steps to alleviate the problem without medication or other treatments?

✓ Keep in mind that sometimes better and more affordable health care is *less* health care. But sometimes delaying treatment can make the problem worse or more expensive to treat—for example, if you end up in the emergency room on a weekend. So be ready to see your doctor right away for problems that could be potentially serious or could develop into a worse problem without attention (like out-of-control asthma; a sudden, unusual, and severe headache; severe injury; or signs of a heart attack or stroke).

4

Don't Pay for Chronic Diseases . . . Avoid Them!

L ike an endless stream of armored cars stuffed with cash, a great deal of America's healthcare dollars flows toward covering chronic conditions.

Our nation spends 84 percent of its healthcare dollars on people with chronic conditions, according to a 2010 report from the Robert Wood Johnson Foundation. Half of all Americans who aren't living in institutions such as a nursing home have a chronic condition, and more than one-quarter of Americans have at least two of these conditions. Nearly half of those with a chronic condition have multiple conditions.

Developing a chronic illness or other serious health problem can have a sizable impact on your household finances. For example:

🖤 People with diagnosed diabetes have medical expenses that are an estimated 2.3 times higher than if they didn't have diabetes. As a result, having diabetes might set you back an average of $6,649 extra each year, according to a 2008 article in *Diabetes Care.*

🖤 Patients with cardiovascular disease have more than twice the medical costs of people the same age without cardio-vascular disease. A 2010 study in the *American Journal of Managed Care* followed more than 12,000 patients with cardiovascular disease and found that, on average, they had nearly $19,000 in total annual medical costs.

🖤 A 2009 study found that being actively treated for can-cer runs patients an average of $1,170 in higher out-of-pocket medical expenses each year, and is associated with a greater risk of not being employed full-time. In 2006, nearly a quarter of insured adults whose households had been affected by cancer said they'd run through most or all of their savings during treatment. Another study, this one from 2010, found that nearly 8 percent of cancer survivors went without medical care, nearly 10 percent went without medications, and more than 11 percent went without dental care because of the cost. As a result, the researchers estimated that more than 2 million cancer survivors in America from 2003 to 2006 didn't get at least one medical service they needed due to cost concerns.

🔍 And though it's not technically a disease, obesity raises your risk of many serious chronic health conditions, thus harming your household's bottom line. Obese people have $1,429 higher medical expenses per year than people with a normal weight, according to a 2009 study from the journal *Health Affairs.* The authors also write that obesity is associated with 9.1 percent of overall annual medical spending nationwide, a percentage that has increased in recent years and is likely to continue to increase.

If you want to enjoy better health and keep more money in your pocket—and less flowing into the healthcare system in coming years—it's crucial that you protect yourself from chronic diseases. In the end, much of this responsibility comes down to you. The decisions you make, day in and day out, largely shape your risk of some of the most common chronic diseases, many of which are almost entirely preventable. Others may not be preventable per se, but you can still have an impact on reducing your risk.

Although your doctor can help, you're going to have to do much of the work to help lower your risk of these diseases. Changes that you can make in your life can have a very real impact on whether or not you'll develop a major illness. Avoiding the preventable risk factors that can lead to illness doesn't just save you money, of course: it can add years to your life and improve the quality of all the years you have coming, as well.

According to a 2009 study in the journal *PLoS Medicine*, in 2005 an estimated:

467,000 deaths were due to tobacco smoking

395,000 were due to high blood pressure

216,000 were due to being overweight or obese

191,000 were due to physical inactivity

190,000 were due to high blood sugar

102,000 were due to diets high in salt

82,000 were due to diets high in trans-fatty acids

64,000 were due to alcohol use

Not convinced that your behaviors are directly related to whether or not you'll develop a condition that could seriously affect your quality of life and cost you a lot of money? We can keep going.

Research suggests that 80 percent of the cases of diabetes, heart disease, and stroke in this country could be prevented simply by eliminating tobacco use and reducing obesity. According to the American Cancer Society, about 188,000 of the cancer deaths that occurred in 2010 were related to being overweight or obese, having a physically inactive lifestyle, or eating an unhealthy diet. About 171,000 cancer deaths were caused by tobacco use.

Although you've probably heard the refrain of "don't smoke, get more exercise, and watch your weight" many times, it's important to remember that these sensible approaches don't just keep you healthier in some distant future that you can worry about later.

Making smart lifestyle choices can also mean the difference between enjoying good *financial* health and spending thousands of dollars on preventable illnesses. By staying healthier, you may need less sick days away from work. You may feel better during the day and enjoy more productivity. You also might avoid early disability that would reduce your earning potential. Improving your lifestyle is economical in a different way, too. You don't have to make a bunch of separate changes to lower your risk of diabetes, heart disease, stroke, cancer, and other diseases. In many cases, the same small number of steps will help protect you from multiple conditions.

In this chapter, we'll discuss why you should develop a disease-preventing lifestyle . . . and how you can do so.

In 2008, the Agency for Healthcare Research and Quality listed the ten most expensive medical conditions. We'll provide tips on preventing some of the big-ticket illnesses on their list: heart conditions, cancer, high blood pressure, and type 2 diabetes. We'll also touch on dementia here, and in the next chapter we'll provide tips on preventing other common medical problems.

✦ ✦ ✦

Preventing Diabetes-Related Expenses

In 2007, diabetes set America back at least $116 billion in direct medical costs and $58 billion for other costs, such as disability and lost work time, according to the American Diabetes

Association. Each year, 1.6 million adults are diagnosed with diabetes, which is more than the population of Dallas, Texas.

When we talk about diabetes here, we're referring to the most common kind: type 2 diabetes. Type 1 diabetes is a disease in which your immune system attacks cells in your pancreas. It usually occurs earlier in life and is not typically regarded as preventable.

Why are we putting diabetes first on our list of expensive chronic conditions you should avoid? Three reasons. The first is that diabetes can serve as the first teetering domino that sets off a cascade of expensive medical events. Complications of diabetes include cardiovascular disease, blindness, kidney disease, erectile dysfunction, gum disease, and slow-healing injuries on the feet that can lead to the need for amputation. This can fuel a lot of expenses for medications, surgeries, and other treatments, as well as time away from work and reduced quality of life.

The second reason we're starting with diabetes is that it's largely preventable through lifestyle changes. A 2009 study published in the *Archives of Internal Medicine* that followed nearly 5,000 men and women ages sixty-five and older for ten years found that 90 percent of new cases of diabetes appeared to be due to a handful of lifestyle factors: physical activity, diet, smoking, alcohol use, and body size. If participants fell into the low-risk group for all of these factors, they had an 89 percent lower risk of developing diabetes.

And a third reason to make a priority of avoiding the expense of diabetes is that the basic preventive steps—not smoking, watching your diet, avoiding obesity, and getting enough physical activity—are the fundamental steps for avoiding many other big, expensive diseases. Though we just mentioned a study that included older people with diabetes, people should be concerned about this disease at a much younger age. In 2000, the average age at diagnosis for type 2 diabetes was forty-six, according to research published in the *Annals of Family Medicine* in 2005. In addition, your doctor may find signs that your body is headed toward diabetes years before it develops.

If you want to avoid this pricey disorder, don't wait to start worrying about it when you're in your forties or beyond. Whatever your age, start now. If an ounce of prevention is worth a pound of cure, then a few pennies of prevention can save you thousands of dollars of treatment and a much-reduced quality of life. Following are the essential methods for avoiding diabetes, according to the National Diabetes Information Clearinghouse.

Keep your body weight at a normal level. You probably know the rules of healthy living by now. After all, we've heard them many times from our moms, our teachers, billboards, TV commercials, and our kids' science-fair projects. In theory, they seem like great ideas that we know are somehow good for us. But when we're living our lives day to day, these guidelines may not seem as compelling.

However, healthy behaviors have very real and specific effects inside our bodies. It's like how wearing a seat belt isn't good for your health because of some abstract, hard-to-imagine explanation. It works by keeping you from hurting your vital organs or flying out of the car during a wreck.

In the same way, keeping your weight at a healthy level isn't just some good idea in theory. It's the condition your body *needs* to be in if it's going to work properly. **If you're overweight, quite a few expensive and unwanted outcomes are more likely to happen.** In terms of diabetes, your body's cells run on sugar, called glucose. Your pancreas produces a hormone called insulin, which allows your cells to bring in the glucose and use it for fuel. A problem called "insulin resistance"—in which insulin doesn't act on your cells like it should—is how type 2 diabetes usually begins.

Having too much fat in your body plays an important role in insulin resistance. Fat isn't just a neutral substance that you carry around like a pillow stuffed under your shirt. It's an active tissue that releases chemicals that can affect whether your body's cells are sensitive to insulin or resistant to it. Body fat appears especially hazardous to your insulin sensitivity when it builds up deep in your abdomen (known as visceral fat), as opposed to the squishy layer just beneath your skin.

If glucose doesn't get into your cells where it's supposed to be, it can build up in your blood circulation. A chronically high level can damage your blood vessels and nerves, setting the stage for complications. Your pancreas may try harder to get your cells to work by producing even more insulin, which can tire it out and leave it unable to keep up its production.

So when it comes to preventing diabetes, shedding extra pounds is a good place to start. You don't have to get model-skinny to reduce your risk. The American Diabetes Association points out that losing just 7 percent of your weight can help. For someone who weighs 200 pounds, that would be 14 pounds. If you need some guidance on what a healthy weight would be for your height, figure out your body mass index (BMI). You'll find a BMI chart on page 130–131. In general, a healthy range is 18.5 to 24.9.

Being especially muscular can make your number high (and overestimate your health risk), but in general, if your BMI's between 25 and 29.9, you're considered overweight, and it's wise to consider bringing your weight down. Obesity begins at 30 and above. Measuring your waist is also a quick way to see if your weight may be putting you at risk. In a 2007 study in *Diabetes Care*, researchers found that when nearly 6,000 people were divided into three groups, those in the medium and high waist circumference groups were more likely to have diabetes. If you're a woman, aim for a waist circumference below 35 inches; men should aim for less than 40 inches.

You'll find plenty of good reasons to lose weight, but since this book is looking at the financial implications of poor health, let's take into account the dollar cost of being too heavy. In a 2008 article in the journal *Obesity,* researchers estimated the costs that come with being overweight or obese. They calculated that for twenty-year-olds who have crossed over into obesity, lifetime costs due to their weight are $16,490 and $12,290 for white and black men, respectively, and $21,550 and $5,340 for white and black women, respectively. The costs are even higher for severely obese individuals.

As the authors point out, even if joining a gym costs several hundred dollars a year, if it helps keep you from becoming obese, it might be a money-saving investment.

Eat a sensible diet. A word that largely sums up the diet that can help prevent diabetes is *fiber*. The American Diabetes Association recommends that people at high risk of diabetes eat 14 grams of fiber for every 1,000 calories they consume. For a 2,000-calorie diet, that would be 28 grams of fiber, or about what you'd find in one-half cup of black beans, plus a cup of raspberries, plus a cup of raisin bran. But even if you're *not* at high risk of diabetes, a high-fiber diet is also a reasonable step to take, since getting adequate fiber has been linked to lower LDL cholesterol and a reduced risk of heart disease. It has also been linked to a reduced risk of certain cancers.

A diet that provides more fiber tends to be rich in fruits, vegetables, beans, and whole grains. Making even relatively small changes in the foods you eat can make a big impact on your diabetes risk. In a June 2010 study from the *Archives of Internal Medicine*, researchers found that people who ate at least five servings of white rice a week had a 17 percent higher risk of type 2 diabetes than those who ate it less than once a month. However, those who ate at least two servings of *brown* rice weekly had an 11 percent lower risk of diabetes than those who ate it less than once a month.

Another 2010 study published in the journal *BMJ* honed in on fruit and vegetable consumption effects on type 2 diabetes. More than 220,000 participants were included across six studies.

The researchers found that eating just one and a half extra servings of green leafy vegetables each day reduced the risk of type 2 diabetes by 14 percent. The authors suggested that this protective effect was due, at least in part, to antioxidants and possibly specific nutrients (such as the magnesium in spinach and other green, leafy vegetables).

A diabetes-preventing diet is also relatively low in fat. According to the National Diabetes Information Clearinghouse, fat should account for no more than one-quarter of your daily calories, which means if you're aiming for, say, 1,600 calories daily, you wouldn't want more than 44 grams of fat (which contains nine calories per gram).

People often claim that healthy natural foods—like fruits and vegetables—cost more than processed foods. Indeed, this may be true. And it may be an issue that's growing worse. A 2007 study in the *Journal of the American Dietetic Association* looked at costs of 372 foods and beverages in Seattle supermarkets in 2004 and 2006. Over this period, the cost of foods that were lowest in energy density (which are generally the healthy foods you want) went up by nearly 20 percent. The most energy-dense foods (which are typically less desirable for health) went *down* in cost by nearly 2 percent.

However, don't get caught in the trap of thinking that cheaper is better at the supermarket. If you figure in the future health costs that are hidden away in the fatty, sugary, salty foods that are so common in the American diet, these really don't seem like good deals after all. Take extra time to look for bargains in your supermarket, like bags of dried beans, slow-cook brown rice in bulk, and nuts in the shell. Check out your local farmers market during the summer. Clip coupons and watch for sales. And if you find that you need to cut back on fast food, sodas, candy bars, beer, and cigarettes in order to prevent expensive diseases, apply the money you're saving toward buying more nutritious foods.

Stay physically active. A landmark study from 2002 investigated just how useful lifestyle changes are for preventing type 2 diabetes. All the participants were overweight and had prediabetes, which put them squarely in the path of diabetes. Some were given intensive counseling on how to improve their lifestyle, with the goal of losing 7 percent of their body weight. Some were given the insulin-sensitizing drug metformin, while a third group merely received placebo pills. Those in the metformin and placebo groups received information about diet and exercise but weren't offered the intensive motivational counseling.

The researchers found that after about three years, people who attempted to lose 7 percent of their body weight by cutting back on calories and exercising for 150 minutes weekly cut their risk of developing diabetes by more than half compared with the placebo group. In comparison, the people who took metformin lowered their risk by 31 percent compared to those receiving a placebo.

Another study from 2009 in the *Lancet* discussed what happened to these participants in the following years. All the groups were offered the lifestyle intervention, and most of the people taking metformin continued to do so. During the follow-up study, rates of new diabetes cases were similar in all the groups. But the rate of diabetes in the lifestyle group was 34 percent lower compared to the placebo group—suggesting that the effect of lifestyle changes on preventing or delaying diabetes can last for at least ten years.

Exercise not only helps you stay at a healthy weight, it also improves your insulin sensitivity, because *moving* is what your body really wants. Think of your body as a well-crafted machine. This machine needs certain maintenance to run properly. The machinery of the body was designed to function as an active machine. It *needs* to move in order to stay tuned up and fully functional. When left idle, problems arise and the machine begins to shut down. Muscles start to dwindle, and pounds start to pile on. Instead of being a lean, mean, fightin' machine, you start to become lethargic, slow, weak, and increasingly unhappy. Your body simply doesn't work properly when it's set on idle. It leads to pounds of extra fat that are pumping out disruptive chemicals, slowing the machine down further.

The modern lifestyle that so many Americans lead—in which we drive wherever we need to go, do many of our jobs by sitting at a phone or computer, and have machines and devices that do much of our manual labor for us—simply doesn't require our bodies to work as they were built to function. For thousands of years, people's bodies most often took in fuel then burned it off. They didn't take it in and find a place to store the excess year after year.

And our bodies need *steady* amounts of exercise. It's great if you're getting a thirty-minute workout at the gym most days a week. But that should be your *starting* point. If you can safely walk or bike to the grocery store, bank, or post office, leave the car at home. If you have an hour to spend on TV on a warm summer evening, leave it off and go outside for a walk or a session throwing the baseball back and forth with your child. Walk on your lunch hour. Walk to a coworker's office instead of sending e-mails. Buy a $10 pedometer for your belt and see how high you can raise that number of steps every day (many experts recommend aiming for 10,000 steps a day).

Whatever you do, just keep moving. It will pay off. A Canadian study from a 2009 issue of *Health Economics* estimated that a person who is inactive spends 38 percent more days in the hospital, makes 5.5 percent more visits to the family physician, and uses 13 percent more specialist services than someone who is active.

See your doctor. Your doctor can test you for a condition called prediabetes, which is marked by high blood sugar levels that don't quite meet the standard for diabetes. The Diabetes Prevention Program study discussed earlier found that about 11 percent of people with prediabetes who were in the placebo group went on to develop full-blown diabetes each year over a three-year period. Your doctor can also check you for other threats to your heart health, like high blood pressure and high cholesterol, which often go hand in hand with high blood sugar.

Your primary care doctor—who hopefully will find out soon that you're trying to avoid costly conditions—can make suggestions on how to change your diet and physical activity patterns based on your unique needs, which may give you an extra spark of motivation. Remember: people with prediabetes around the world are keeping themselves from getting diabetes. A Finnish study found that lifestyle changes significantly reduced people's risk, with benefits lasting for years afterward. A Chinese study also found a lower risk of type 2 diabetes after six years from a lifestyle intervention. You can do it too.

Your doctor can also recommend several medications that have been shown to reduce the risk of full-blown diabetes in people with prediabetes. Just keep in mind that medications usually cost money, and they may have side effects. Physical activity and eating healthier (or at least cutting out the *un*healthy stuff) cost little, and they protect you from many diseases, not just diabetes.

Preventing Cardiovascular Disease- and Stroke-Related Expenses

Cardiovascular diseases and stroke cost the United States an estimated $475 billion in 2009, according to the American Heart Association (AHA). Fueling these costs is a constant stream of heart attacks and strokes across the nation. Every twenty-five seconds, someone has a coronary event, such as a heart attack. Every forty seconds, someone has a stroke.

Many of the same protective strategies that will help protect you from diabetes will also help to ensure that you don't have to suffer the great expense and likelihood of lost income due to heart disease or a stroke. For starters, simply avoiding diabetes can help keep you safe from heart disease and stroke. Research published in the *Lancet* found that diabetes may *double* your risk of diseases like heart disease or stroke.

Nine percent of adult American men and 7 percent of women have coronary heart disease, also known as coronary artery disease, according to the AHA. This condition is due to buildup of a blend of cholesterol, fat, and other substances in the walls of the arteries feeding your heart muscle. Healthy coronary arteries, by the way, are only fractions of a centimeter across, so they don't have a lot of room for things to go bad. Your heart demands a steady flow of nutrients and oxygen through these small vessels to support it as it beats away day after day. If these vessels grow narrow, your heart may have a painful reaction called angina. If the blood flow becomes blocked, such as from a blood clot in an already narrowed vessel, it causes a heart attack.

Coronary artery disease can also lead to heart failure. When this occurs, your heart simply can't pump blood out to your body as well as it should. Heart failure affects an estimated 5 million Americans, and research has found it to be one of the most expensive chronic illnesses in adults. Most hospitalizations and deaths related to heart failure occur in people who are sixty-five and older. About two-thirds of the costs of heart failure are due to hospitalizations. The rest are for expenses such as doctor's visits, trips to the ER, and medications.

A condition that is often discussed alongside heart disease is stroke. More than 600,000 Americans have a first stroke every year, and every four minutes, someone dies of one, according to the AHA. The most common kind of stroke has a lot in common with a heart attack: The flow of blood through an artery feeding the brain becomes blocked, and an area of brain tissue becomes starved for fuel and oxygen. A less-common type of stroke is caused by a blood vessel that bleeds into the brain.

A 2006 study found that the cost of an ischemic stroke—the common kind in which blood flow is cut off—was $15,597 for whites, $17,201 for Hispanics, and $25,782 for African Americans. Why do strokes cost more for some groups than others? The answer reminds us of yet another reason why it's in our best financial interest to keep from getting sick, regardless of whether or not we have good insurance.

The researchers added in more than just the direct costs of medical care, and one of the *indirect* costs they included was the largest factor in overall costs: lost earnings. Strokes are a common cause of disability in the United States. Hispanics and African Americans tend to have strokes at an earlier age than whites, thus they lose more of their potential to earn an income. Another major cost was for informal caregiving, like family members providing care when they could be working.

Many of the conditions in this chapter and Chapter 5 have the potential to keep you away from work, either for a short period or a long time. Clearly, as you're making changes to slash medical expenses, doing what you can to sidestep heart disease and strokes offers big money-saving opportunities. According to the AHA, you can take many steps to protect yourself:

Know your risk. The AHA recommends that you start working with your doctor to learn your risk of heart disease starting at age twenty. You should have your lipids (also known as cholesterol) and blood sugar tested at least every five years, and possibly every two years if you're at higher risk. All adults older than forty should also know their overall risk of developing coronary artery disease, the organization urges. The goal? Getting this risk score as low as possible. It's a good idea to figure out your risk with your doctor, but if you'd like to get a sense of what kind of threat you face from a heart attack, you can find a quiz through the National Institutes of Health at http://hp2010.nhlbihin.net/atpiii/calculator.asp, or search online for the words Framingham Heart Risk Calculator.

Stop smoking and avoid secondhand smoke. Smoking is simply not a good idea, either from a health or personal-finance standpoint. Your risk of heart disease is doubled or even quadrupled when you smoke, according to the AHA. Given that heart disease is already so common for people in general, smoking puts you at major risk of heart problems.

This is probably not new information to you. But this book is about getting the best health for your buck, so let's talk about what a pack of cigarettes *really* costs you. Let's say you're paying $5 a pack, though they cost far more in many areas. At just one pack a day, that's $1,825 each year. That could cover one or more mortgage payments, or your car payments for several months.

If you're a thirty-five-year-old smoker and started investing this money at 6 percent interest, you'd have more than $160,000 at age sixty-five. Of course, cigarettes will cost more in the future than whatever you're paying now, so you'd have even more pay-off if you put your smoking money into an investment.

However, let's not pretend that the money you pay at the register is the *only* price you'll pay for those cigarettes. Smoking in your car can lower its resale value. The same goes for your home. Some companies prefer to not *hire* smokers. According to media reports in 2010, a Tennessee hospital began refusing to hire people who smoked, even in their spare time. (Even dry-cleaning your clothes and having a mint won't hide a smoking habit at a job interview, since a urine test easily shows if you smoke.) In today's tough job market, why put yourself at any potential disadvantage? Need more reasons? Life insurance can cost a lot more if you smoke. Your health insurance premiums may cost more, too.

Over the years, a number of researchers have estimated what a pack of cigarettes *really* costs once you figure in the illnesses and early death that tend to befall people who smoke. A 2008 study from the *Journal of Health Economics* concluded that the cost of the early loss of life equals $222 per pack for men and $94 per pack for women. The cost is higher for men than women, according to the authors, since smoking has a bigger impact on mortality for men, and they also tend to earn higher wages. This study involved a lot of statistical juggling, and previous studies had calculated the hidden costs of smoking to be much less per pack—but still a lot more than the price you pay at the register.

Quitting smoking is tough. If it weren't, fewer people would still be smoking. We're not really expecting you to smack your forehead and say, "Hey, smoking's expensive! I'm going to quit this minute now that I know this!" Your desire for that cigarette *now* can be a lot more compelling than an illness—or a bigger retirement account—years down the road. But just remember that you make many other decisions today in the hopes that they'll improve your situation in some distant future. When you're looking for a new home, you probably include its potential resale value in your decision. You may go back to school for another degree in the hopes of a better job years from now. You set money aside in a 401(k) instead of buying something fun now. You can look at your habits related to smoking, eating, and exercising the same way.

If you're not ready to quit now, think about when you might want to quit. Six months from now? A year from now? What are the issues and reasons that are prompting you to keep smoking now? How could you start working through those so they no longer compel you to smoke? When you're closer to being ready to quit, get your doctor involved in helping you. Your doctor can recommend or prescribe nicotine replacement products and medications that can improve your ability to stop smoking. The short-term cost of the successful use of any of these will be smaller than the price of continuing the habit. Also, check out whether your employer offers any resources or incentives to help you stop smoking. Try to find someone else who's successfully quit, and ask for advice and encouragement.

As far as secondhand smoke goes, perhaps it's best to think about it as one of the names the American Cancer Society gives it: involuntary smoking. Someone else is choosing to smoke, but *you're* breathing in nicotine and toxins. Involuntary smoking can contribute to the development of cancer, heart disease, lung infections, and—in children—ear infections and more frequent asthma attacks. If you see someone lighting up, head in the other direction or ask them to smoke elsewhere. Why should you pay a possible price for someone else's smoking?

Keep your weight down. According to the AHA, being overweight increases your risk of coronary heart disease by raising your blood pressure, reducing your "good" HDL cholesterol, and contributing to diabetes.

More than 50 million Americans are thought to have a cluster of health problems that combine to create "metabolic syndrome." These include obesity (especially around the belly), harmful lipids that promote plaque buildup in artery walls (that is, low HDL and high LDL cholesterol and triglycerides), high blood pressure, trouble properly handling insulin or blood sugar, and high levels of inflammatory chemicals. Metabolic syndrome puts you at higher risk of coronary heart disease, diabetes, and stroke.

The lifestyle changes that promote weight loss are largely free or low in cost: get more physical activity (at least thirty minutes on most days), clean up your diet (more on that in a moment), and strive to get your body mass index below 25.

If you're significantly overweight, keep in mind that the benefits of weight loss for heart disease aren't all-or-nothing. The protection doesn't wait to kick in only when your body mass index is below 25. According to the AHA, losing as little as ten pounds can help you avoid developing heart disease.

Losing weight and keeping it off doesn't typically happen through fad diets or by making one big, sweeping change. It comes from changing the way you think about how you eat and how you use your free time. It comes from making a bundle of tiny changes until your life is headed in a different direction fitnesswise. Check out Chapter 7 on developing a mind-set that helps you make these changes.

Eat like the Mediterraneans do. Eating a diet that helps you prevent disease isn't something you do just one time. Nor do you get the benefits by eating a particular meal once a week. If you want to stay healthy in the coming years and keep your money in your pocket and out of the healthcare system, you need to make reasonable choices day after day, year after year, and decade after decade.

As a result, you're going to need to find a style of eating that appeals to you for the long term. Fad diets are by their nature virtually impossible to stick with. Forcing yourself to eat foods you don't like isn't going to work, either. And completely eliminating your favorites is no way to live your life. A better way to go may be to simply pattern your eating habits after the Mediterranean diet.

This doesn't mean eating in Greek and Italian restaurants (though you can certainly do so). Instead, a Mediterranean-type diet means that your meals and snacks are largely composed of:

- 🐚 Fruits and vegetables
- 🐚 Whole-grain bread and other whole-grain foods
- 🐚 Beans, seeds, and nuts

As part of this diet, you also eat seafood several times a week but not much red meat. Much of your fat comes from olive oil, which is rich in desirable monounsaturated fat. Salt is used sparingly. This eating style makes room for a small amount of alcohol (preferably red wine), if you drink. These food categories provide tons of options to allow you to create meals that satisfy your own tastes and assemble a diet that you can stick with for decades. The research supporting the Mediterranean diet as a tool for fighting many diseases continues to pour in.

One 2008 study from the journal *BMJ* compiled the results of twelve earlier studies that involved more than 1.5 million people who were followed for at least three years. People who more closely stuck with a Mediterranean-type diet were 9 percent less likely to die in general and 9 percent less likely to die of a cardiovascular condition. They were also less likely to develop cancer or Alzheimer's disease, which we'll be talking about later in this chapter.

Another study, published in the journal *Circulation* in August 2010, suggested that eating a lot of red meat raises the risk of coronary heart disease. After following more than 84,000 women, the researchers found that having a serving of nuts per day compared to red meat was linked to a 30 percent lower risk of coronary heart disease. A daily serving of low-fat dairy, poultry, and fish were linked to 13, 19, and 24 percent lower risks, respectively, compared to red meat.

Drink lightly—if you drink at all. Alcohol may play different roles in cardiovascular disease, depending on how much you drink. Drinking a small amount—up to one drink daily for women or up to two drinks for men—is actually associated with lower risk of heart disease.

Two studies from a March 2010 *Journal of the American College of Cardiology* offered more support for alcohol and heart protection. In one, the researchers pooled the results of eight previous studies featuring more than 16,000 people with a history of cardiovascular disease. Light to moderate alcohol use was associated with reduced risk of death, either from any cause or from cardiovascular causes. In the other study, the researchers reviewed national health-related surveys of a representative sample of American adults. Light drinkers had a 31 percent lower chance of dying of heart-related issues, and moderate drinkers had a 38 percent lower chance, compared to people who never drank. If you're going to drink alcohol, red wine may be a particularly good choice for heart health.

However, drinking an excessive amount can raise your risk of high blood pressure and stroke. Alcohol also raises the risk of a variety of cancers, and even having a few drinks a week over the long term can raise a woman's breast cancer risks.

Get enough physical activity. As we said earlier in the diabetes section, the time you spend on your feet getting physical activity on most days helps prevent many diseases at one time. According to the AHA, physical activity helps prevent or lower high blood pressure, insulin resistance, high triglycerides and bad LDL cholesterol, and obesity, and it helps boost your good HDL cholesterol.

At the risk of sounding like a late-night infomercial, how much would you pay for a pill that could provide all those improvements? You can get the benefits of physical activity for little to no money—just put on a pair of shoes and go for a walk or play in the yard with your kids. Get at least thirty minutes on most or all days—with an emphasis on *at least*. Physical activity isn't some obscure thing that should be a hassle to fit into your day. It's a basic requirement that your body needs just like food, water, and sleep. Your body, that intricately designed machine, depends on it.

Yoga may be a particularly helpful form of exercise to add to a regimen for people concerned about maintaining their heart health. It's meditative, it can improve your flexibility, and some research suggests that it may be helpful for reducing elevated blood pressure and improving heart failure outcomes.

Keep tabs on your mental and emotional health. Evidence suggests that mood and emotional issues—such as depression and anger—may threaten your heart health. In a 2004 study in the *Archives of Internal Medicine* that followed nearly 94,000 women, depression in women without a history of cardiovascular disease was associated with a 50 percent higher risk of cardiovascular-related death. Another study in the *European Heart Journal* found that people who more often expressed positive emotions had a 22 percent lower risk of coronary heart disease. Symptoms of depression also predicted coronary heart disease. Other research points to poorer outcomes in people who chronically suppress their anger.

The association between depression and other emotional factors with heart disease is drawing a lot of research attention these days, and it appears likely that these problems are important factors that can put you at risk. If you feel that stress, anxiety, depression, or poorly controlled anger is a problem for you, talk to your doctor or a mental health practitioner about ways to cope with these issues. Self-help steps that may be helpful include exercise and meditation.

Take care of your teeth. Experts have put quite a bit of focus in recent years on exploring the links between oral health and heart health. If you don't take good care of your teeth and gums, you can get infection and inflammation in your gums, which in turn can raise levels of inflammatory chemicals throughout your body. These, in turn, can cause damage in your blood vessels, which can contribute to heart disease. It's like a row of dominos that starts at your teeth and leads to your chest.

A 2010 study that involved nearly 12,000 middle-aged and older Scottish adults found that those who brushed their teeth less than once a day had a 70 percent higher risk of cardiovascular disease-related problems compared to those who brushed twice a day. The American Dental Association recommends twice-daily brushing, as well as cleaning between your teeth daily with floss or an interdental cleaner. Spending a little time with a brush and floss each day seems like a no-brainer, an easy—and inexpensive—way to protect yourself from an incredibly expensive ailment.

Take medications as necessary. Statins and blood pressure drugs are commonly prescribed these days, and you and your doctor may conclude that you need one or more of these drugs if your cholesterol or hypertension is putting your heart at risk. But before you start taking these, remember to ask your doctor the questions we discussed in Chapter 3:

- Why do I need these?
- Can I make any changes on my own that will keep me from having to take these? (Be ready for the talk about diet, exercise, not smoking, and losing weight that we just discussed—but which will be given more quickly.)
- Which of my drug options will work the best for the lowest price?
- What side effects should I watch for?
- What follow-up will this treatment require, such as regular office visits or blood tests?
- Can we set goals that, if reached, will allow me to discontinue these medications at some point?

Drugs for lowering your cholesterol or high blood pressure are intended to be used for a long time. If you stop taking them—which many people do—they stop working for you. Our goal is for people to reduce their disease risk on their own to avoid the expense of medications. But if you and your doctor decide that you *do* need a drug, then your goal should become using it as effectively as possible. But remember that taking medications isn't always a lifetime commitment. You can work to get yourself off medications for many chronic conditions. Just do so in concert with your doctor to help avoid any pitfalls.

Preventing Cancer-Related Expenses

Cancer soaked up about $264 billion worth of American resources in 2010, according to the American Cancer Society, quoting figures from the National Institutes of Health. Of this, $103 billion was for direct medical costs, such as surgeries, medications, and other treatments. Another $21 billion or so came from the cost of people not being able to work because they were sick. And more than $140 billion was due to loss of productivity from people dying too soon.

According to a study by researchers from the American Cancer Society announced in August 2010, cancer has the most significant economic impact of any cause of death worldwide. In 2008, the disease led to nearly one *trillion* dollars in economic losses from early death and disability, which doesn't count the direct medical costs of treating cancer.

Given that more than 1.5 million Americans are diagnosed with cancer on an annual basis these days—and this is our second-leading cause of death in America—it's worth considering what you're willing to do in order to avoid cancer.

If cancer were to make an appearance in your life, it could make a huge impact on your household's finances and your family's peace of mind. And if it strikes you while you're still working, it could affect your job.

A 2009 study of more than 89,000 people of working age found that those actively undergoing care for cancer missed about twenty-two more days of work per year than people without cancer. Symptoms of cancer or side effects of treatment—including pain, fatigue, and difficulty concentrating—can also affect your ability to focus at work. The Americans with Disabilities Act offers some protections to employees with cancer, but the disease can still be very disruptive to your job. And if you're one of the millions of Americans who are self-employed—like this book's coauthor Eric—an inability to work could quickly become disastrous.

Finally, if you were to die of cancer, how would the loss of your income affect your family's future? Cancer tends to occur late in one's career or in retirement. But plenty of people have it in their prime income-earning years. One-third of breast cancer cases are diagnosed between the ages of thirty-five and fifty-four, according to recent statistics from the National Cancer Institute. More than one-quarter of cases of cancer of the mouth and pharynx (throat) are also diagnosed during this time. And nearly 40 percent of melanoma cases are diagnosed under the age of fifty-five.

The thought of getting cancer isn't fun to consider. And as with the other diseases we're talking about here, it can be hard to base your day-to-day decisions on the hope of avoiding a scary outcome years or even decades from now. But as we said earlier, we make choices all the time that we hope will pay off in the distant future. And not having cancer is a good payoff.

The list of steps that will help you reduce your risk of cancer includes many of the same ideas that will protect you from the other diseases mentioned in this chapter. But please keep reading even if you feel like you've heard enough of the whole "healthy living" message already. Knowing about all the money-saving (and lifesaving) benefits that you can obtain for free or little expense may help keep you motivated to make smart changes and stick with them.

Don't smoke or use other tobacco products. When you smoke or use smokeless tobacco products, you're paying a big business a sizable chunk of your hard-earned income for a product that very well could kill you. Tobacco use accounts for at least one-third of cancer deaths, according to the American Cancer Society (ACS). And tobacco use is an entirely preventable risk factor for cancer. If you smoke or chew, you're going *out of your way* to stand directly in the path of cancer of the mouth, lungs, stomach, larynx, throat, kidneys, bladder, and other body parts.

Cancer and other diseases from tobacco use can leave your savings account empty and leave you unable to work. They can leave you gasping for air while doing simple tasks. They can leave you disfigured and disabled. If you're still buying cigarettes or other tobacco products, maybe it's finally time to leave *them*. More than 48 million Americans have stopped smoking. You can do it, too.

Limit your exposure to ultraviolet (UV) rays. About 70,000 cases of melanoma were diagnosed in 2010, and more than 2 million people were treated for basal and squamous skin cancer in 2006. Melanoma is a particularly dangerous form of skin cancer, and it accounts for about three-quarters of annual skin-cancer deaths.

Even though nonmelanoma cancers such as basal and squamous cell carcinoma may be less threatening to your health, getting them removed from your skin can also take a chunk out of your bank account. A 2009 article from the *Journal of the American Academy of Dermatology* found a wide range of costs associated with getting a basal cell carcinoma removed from the cheek or a squamous cell carcinoma removed from the forearm. Treatments ranged from about $400 for removal of the forearm cancer with an electrical device to more than $3,000 to excise the cheek cancer in a hospital operating room.

Preventing skin cancer, however, is very inexpensive. According to the ACS, the best methods to lower your risk are to:

- Limit your exposure to the sun, especially between 10:00 AM and 4:00 PM.
- Wear a wide-brimmed hat, sunglasses that block UV A and B rays, and long-sleeved shirts and long pants or skirts with tightly woven fabric.
- Before heading out into the sun, apply a thick layer of sunscreen with an SPF of 30 or higher to any exposed skin. Be sure the product hasn't expired; sunscreen usu-

ally works for at least two or three years, according to the ACS. Reapply it every two hours, or more frequently if you're swimming or sweating heavily. A common pitfall is that people don't use enough product; a guideline to follow is using a palmful to cover the average adult's arms, legs, neck, and face.

🗨 Avoid indoor tanning beds and sunlamps.

Eat a cancer-fighting diet. In its 2006 guidelines, the ACS recommends an easy-to-remember diet for cancer prevention. Ready? Eat at least five servings of fruits and vegetables daily, lots of whole grains (like whole-grain bread and pasta) instead of the refined versions, and limit red meat and processed meats. That's it. Of course, some additional tweaks can bring additional benefits.

Some studies have associated a diet high in fiber—in other words, meals and snacks containing fruits and vegetables, beans, and whole grains—with a lower risk of breast and colorectal cancer. When it comes to fruits and vegetables, be sure to eat a variety of choices. In other words, eating potatoes and corn day after day isn't going to work. Some options may be particularly useful against cancer. A diet with lots of cruciferous vegetables, for example, has been linked to a lower risk of lung, bladder, and colorectal cancer. These vegetables include cabbage, broccoli, and Brussels sprouts. One of my favorite (and simple) recipes involves chopping Brussels sprouts, sautéing them in extra virgin olive oil and topping with a bit of sea salt and cracked black pepper. So-called allium vegetables, such as onions and garlic, have also been associated with a lower risk of a variety of cancers.

And a diet rich in tomato products has been linked to a lower risk of prostate cancer, due to the lycopene within them. Cooked tomatoes appear to be a particularly good source of this cancer-fighting warrior, so that's a reason to reach for tomato sauces.

If you're going to have to increase the portion of your food budget that goes toward plant foods, perhaps you can help pay for it by cutting back on meat. A 2009 study in the *Archives of Internal Medicine*, which involved more than half a million people, found that men and women eating the most red meat had about a 21 percent higher risk of dying from cancer than those who ate the least. Those eating the most processed meat had about a 12 percent higher risk of dying from cancer.

Also, if you're going to drink alcohol, limit it to no more than two drinks daily for men, or one for women. A small amount of alcohol may help reduce your risk of cardiovascular disease, but too much alcohol can make you more likely to develop cancer of the mouth, throat, esophagus, liver, or breast.

I see this as using your diet as a preventive tool. We all have to eat. Making smart choices about what we eat at each meal and snack can either work for us or against us. We have several opportunities each day to either boost our health with disease-fighting sustenance or negatively impact our health.

Have you ever noticed that when you go for the sugary, trans-fatty snack or meal choice you crave, you may feel an initial boost, but one that is usually quickly followed by a crash? Have you ever noticed that when you choose a snack or meal that combines a high-quality protein with a complex carbohydrate, you feel satisfied and steadier for longer? This can have a major impact on your daily quality of life and your productivity at work, and over time, these kinds of daily decisions are going to have a major impact on your health.

Keep your weight down. Being overweight or obese may account for 20 percent of all cancer deaths in American women and 14 percent of cancer deaths in men, according to a 2003 study in the *New England Journal of Medicine.*

According to the National Cancer Institute, specific types of cancer that have been associated with obesity include cancer of the colon, breast, endometrium, kidney, and esophagus, and possibly gallbladder, ovarian, and pancreatic cancer. In fact, for breast cancer in postmenopausal women, as well as endometrial, colon, kidney, and esophageal cancer, obesity and lack of physical activity may account for more than a quarter of cases.

It's extremely easy to become overweight in today's world, and more than two-thirds of American adults have done so. More than a third of adults are now obese or heavily overweight. But once again, we see that carrying extra pounds is harmful to your body, setting you up for yet another expensive, painful, and life-altering disease. The effort you put into staying at a healthy weight now—or shedding some extra pounds—can save you a lot of heartache and money later.

Get plenty of exercise. The same minutes that you devote to physical activity in order to reduce your risk of diabetes and heart disease will also help lower your risk of cancer. An extensive body of research has found that physical activity can help protect you from colon cancer, for example. A 2009 study in the *British Journal of Cancer* that compiled the results of fifty-two earlier studies found that being active was associated with a 24 percent lower risk of colon cancer.

Keeping your body physically active may also reduce your risk of breast, endometrial, lung, colon, and prostate cancer, according to the National Cancer Institute. Again, getting at least thirty minutes of moderate-intensity activity on at least five days a week appears to be the *minimum*.

Limit exposure to imaging that uses radiation. X-rays and CT scans are great additions to a healthcare provider's arsenal. These allow your doctor to see what might be going wrong inside your body without putting you through the risk of an invasive surgery in order to look for the problem. But they do expose you to radiation, which carries a cancer risk.

A 2009 study from the *Archives of Internal Medicine* assessed the radiation doses that more than 1,000 patients received while undergoing eleven types of diagnostic CT studies. The radiation doses varied widely depending on the type of CT scan, but the dose for each type of scan also varied between different facilities and even within the same facility. The researchers estimated that one in 270 women who underwent CT coronary angiography at the age of forty—which creates images of the heart's arteries—would develop cancer from the scan. For men, the odds would be one in 600. For twenty-year-old patients, the risks would be roughly doubled, and for sixty-year-old patients, risks would be roughly halved.

This may not sound like a large risk, and in many cases, the benefits of having a scan or x-ray do outweigh this risk. But patients are getting a lot of scans these days, and studies that measure the possible impact of this radiation are now popping up regularly in medical journals. If a medical procedure can raise your risk of cancer (and leave you with additional costs for treating it) by any amount, you'll want to make sure the potential benefits are worth this risk. When a doctor suggests an x-ray or CT scan, ask the questions we suggested in Chapter 3:

- Is this procedure really necessary, or can you get this information some other way that doesn't involve radiation?
- Are the results that you may find from this scan going to change the way you're going to treat this problem?
- Does the potential benefit of this scan outweigh the potential risk?

Be sure to keep track of when you had a scan that uses radiation, and where you received it. It's not uncommon for patients to receive multiple scans that may not be truly necessary while they're traveling around in the healthcare system, due to a lack of communication between their doctors.

Preventing Dementia-Related Expenses

It may be hard to motivate yourself to change your life now in order to protect yourself from dementia, which is a condition in which your brain loses its ability to function properly. After all, dementia—such as Alzheimer's disease—typically occurs in older adults. You may still be decades away from being in an age-group that faces a high risk of dementia.

However, dementia can have a devastating financial impact on you at a time in your life when you can ill-afford the expense. It can leave your spouse in a financially precarious situation and sharply reduce the money you might want to leave your loved ones after a lifetime of hard work and good financial planning.

According to the Alzheimer's Association, 411,000 people were diagnosed with Alzheimer's disease in 2000. That number was expected to rise to more than 450,000 new cases in 2010 and more than 615,000 by 2030. By 2050, that annual number is expected to be just short of 1 million, with someone developing Alzheimer's every thirty-three seconds. Alzheimer's is the most common form of dementia, but another common type is *vascular* dementia, which is typically caused over time by narrowing or blockage of vessels that interrupt blood flow to the brain.

Here's some sobering news from a 2010 Alzheimer's Association report that touches on the many ways dementia can ruin your financial well-being: In 2004, people with dementia in the Medicare program had three times higher Medicare payments than people without dementia. Since that money is coming from someone else, the extra expenses may not be a pressing concern for you, but given our country's aging population, Medicare expenses for dementia could put a strain on the program's abilities to provide for seniors. Something *is* going to give. If you can prepare yourself accordingly, why not do so?

According to the association, the costs of long-term care can quickly grow larger than a typical senior's income. On average, home care costs $152 a day; adult day care costs $67 a day; special dementia care in assisted living facilities is nearly $38,000 a year; and nursing homes run, on average, more than $70,000 a year. One 2005 report from the Kaiser Commission on Medicaid and the Uninsured found that two-thirds of seniors who were still living in the community didn't have enough assets to pay for a year of nursing-home care. People in nursing homes who receive help from Medicaid typically must use most of their income—including Social Security—on their nursing-home care.

The financial impact of dementia can trickle down to following generations. In one study, half of family members and other unpaid caregivers for people with dementia had an average of $219 in caregiving expenses each month, according to the Alzheimer's Association. In addition, adult children and other caregivers may miss out on career advancement opportunities, need to shift to part-time work, or even quit their jobs in order to provide care.

As we've said before, many people spend a lot of time planning and sacrificing *today* to ensure that they have a comfortable retirement. Taking steps to preserve your mental sharpness in your senior years makes at least as much sense. Plus, although dementia typically strikes during one's later years, factors going on in your life now may already be influencing your risk.

Although you may not enjoy the health and financial benefits for decades, the time to act to reduce your risk of dementia is now. Though experts still have a lot to learn about the causes of Alzheimer's and other dementia—and ways to prevent them— these simple steps appear helpful:

Put a taste of the Mediterranean on your plate. We talked about the benefits of the Mediterranean diet earlier in this chapter, and this eating style appears to hold special promise for protecting your brain during your later years.

A 2006 study in the *Annals of Neurology* that followed more than 2,200 older participants found that more than 10 percent of them developed Alzheimer's over an average of four years of follow-up. However, those who most closely stayed with a Mediterranean-type diet had a 40 percent lower risk of Alzheimer's compared to those with the lowest adherence to that type of diet. A 2008 study in the journal *BMJ* compiled the results of twelve earlier studies that included more than 1.5 million people. It found that those who more closely followed a Mediterranean-type diet had a 13 percent lower risk of developing Alzheimer's or Parkinson's.

The Mediterranean diet could help protect you from Alzheimer's (and vascular dementia) in several ways. Damage from free radicals—which are rogue oxygen molecules that can cause harm throughout your body—may play a role in the development of Alzheimer's. The Mediterranean diet provides an abundant supply of antioxidants that can protect you from this damage. Also, inflammation is another problem associated with the development of Alzheimer's, and following this diet may help ease inflammation.

In addition, a diet rich in whole grains, fruits, vegetables, and beans can help lower your cholesterol and blood pressure, thus helping protect against atherosclerosis and strokes that can reduce blood flow to your brain.

Again, the Mediterranean diet includes a lot of whole grains, vegetables, fruits, beans, and olive oil provides much of the fat. It also includes a fair amount of fish, a low to moderate amount of dairy foods, and a bit of wine if you drink. It doesn't, however, include a lot of meat.

Avoid the *other* conditions in this chapter. Like we said at the beginning of this chapter, when you take steps to lower your risk of one chronic condition, you often lower the risk of others. And as you arrive in your later years, your physical health over your lifetime will likely affect your mental abilities.

Many studies have found that older people with diabetes have about twice the risk of dementia or mild cognitive impairment compared to those without diabetes. Obesity in midlife has also been associated with a greater risk of dementia. Additional factors—over which you do have some control—that have been linked with heightened risk of dementia and cognitive decline include high blood pressure and high cholesterol. This is yet another good reason to do what you can to protect yourself from all of these problems.

Keep an eye on depression. Depression, especially late in life, may possibly be associated with a higher risk of dementia. However, researchers aren't sure if the depression leads to the dementia, or if it may simply be an early symptom of dementia.

However, depression may lead to higher levels of the hormone cortisol, which can cause changes in the brain that increase the risk of dementia. People with depression may also have more deposits called beta-amyloid plaques in the brain that are associated with Alzheimer's. You can help keep depression in check with self-help steps including adequate physical activity, but consider getting help from your doctor or mental health professional if depression is a concern in your life.

Avoid tobacco smoke. Research has found a higher risk of dementia in older smokers. Even exposure to other people's smoke may possibly increase your risk. A 2009 study of nonsmokers ages fifty and older found that those with the highest levels of a chemical called cotinine—a marker of exposure to tobacco smoke— were 44 percent more likely to have cognitive impairment.

Stay physically active. Research has found that people who are physically active may have a lower risk of Alzheimer's. Regular physical activity helps keep your blood vessels healthy, which in turn can help protect you from vascular dementia (and may play a role in a lower risk of Alzheimer's). One study found that even four months of exercise can improve people's cognitive ability if they've previously been sedentary.

Keep your brain busy. Some studies have shown that people who participate in activities that involve thinking—like reading or playing games—are less likely to develop dementia. These activities may improve your *cognitive reserve,* sort of like a bank in your mind where you can deposit more resources to have on hand when the passage of time and changes occurring in your brain start making withdrawals. No matter how young or old you are, keep learning. Take a class. Try new hobbies. Learn a musical instrument or foreign language. Do puzzles. Learn something new every day.

Stay socially engaged. On a similar note, people who don't have an active social network also may have a greater risk of developing dementia. Keeping busy with friends and activities outside your home might also improve your cognitive reserve. Plenty of activities and social events are completely free, such as participating in programs at a local library or senior center, volunteering, or taking an active role in senior issues in your community.

Your New Prescription:

✓ Remember that the choices you make every day will help
determine your healthcare costs. Living a healthier life may
not just save you money in the distant future—the savings
may start rapidly.

✓ If you've been thinking about making changes to your life
that will improve your body's ability to work properly without
disease, *now* is the time to start putting those changes into
place. Just four things—eating better, being more physically active, shedding extra pounds, and not smoking—can
save you many thousands of dollars over the course of your
life. Start incorporating small changes into your life that
gradually get you to a healthier lifestyle over the long term
rather than making big changes that are hard to sustain.
Think small changes can't make a difference? Consider the
compound effect we rely on for our retirement accounts:
putting relatively small amounts in over a long time adds up
exponentially. Same applies here, with growing health gains
from small efforts made day in, day out. Over the long term,
your "health portfolio" will be much more robust for your
trouble. Also similar to your retirement account, once you
get into the habit of "sacrificing" the immediate income to
pay yourself first, like anything else, it becomes a habit. In
health changes, this functions exactly the same way.

Body Mass Index Calculator

BMI	19	20	21	22	23	24	25	26	27	28	29	30	31	32	33	34
Height in inches							Body weight in pounds									
58	91	96	100	105	110	115	119	124	129	134	138	143	148	153	158	162
59	94	99	104	109	114	119	124	128	133	138	143	148	153	158	163	168
60	97	102	107	112	118	123	128	133	138	143	148	153	158	163	168	174
61	100	106	111	116	122	127	132	137	143	148	153	158	164	169	174	180
62	104	109	115	120	126	131	136	142	147	153	158	164	169	175	180	186
63	107	113	118	124	130	135	141	146	152	158	163	169	175	180	186	191
64	110	116	122	128	134	140	145	151	157	163	169	174	180	186	192	197
65	114	120	126	132	138	144	150	156	162	168	174	180	186	192	198	204
66	118	124	130	136	142	148	155	161	167	173	179	186	192	198	204	210

Body weight in pounds

BMI	19	20	21	22	23	24	25	26	27	28	29	30	31	32	33	34
Height in inches																
67	121	127	134	140	146	153	159	166	172	178	185	191	198	204	211	217
68	125	131	138	144	151	158	164	171	177	184	190	197	203	210	216	223
69	128	135	142	149	155	162	169	176	182	189	196	203	209	216	223	230
70	132	139	146	153	160	167	174	181	188	195	202	209	216	222	229	236
71	136	143	150	157	165	172	179	186	193	200	208	215	222	229	236	243
72	140	147	154	162	169	177	184	191	199	206	213	221	228	235	242	250
73	144	151	159	166	174	182	189	197	204	212	219	227	235	242	250	257
74	148	155	163	171	179	186	194	202	210	218	225	233	241	249	256	264
75	152	160	168	176	184	192	200	208	216	224	232	240	248	256	264	272
76	156	164	172	180	189	197	205	213	221	230	238	246	254	263	271	279

From National Institutes of Health

5

Preventing Other Common Health Problems

*E*ven though *cancer, heart disease,* and other chronic, life-threatening diseases swallow a substantial portion of our healthcare resources, they're certainly not the only types of illness that can put a dent in your household finances and quality of life.

A lot of the business that goes on in doctors' offices and hospital emergency departments day and night in our country involves issues that developed more acutely, such as infections or accidents, or that are chronic but not life-threatening, like arthritis.

Of course, your health is not completely under your control: Sometimes illnesses and diseases simply happen, and they require intervention from our healthcare system. But as we've seen in the previous chapter, our nation could save billions of dollars every year if more people made more of an effort to sidestep preventable conditions. We've already covered diabetes, heart disease, cancer, and dementia. In this chapter, we'll put the spotlight on some other conditions and problems that add to the charges on many Americans' annual healthcare bills.

Again, you can't always prevent these health issues, but if you try, your effort may be rewarded with better health and big savings on your health care.

✦ ✦ ✦

Preventing Arthritis-Related Expenses

America is becoming an achier place. About one-fifth of all adults have arthritis that was diagnosed by a doctor, according to statistics from the Centers for Disease Control and Prevention (CDC). Half of adults ages sixty-five and older have been diagnosed with arthritis.

The most common kind of arthritis is osteoarthritis, caused by wear and tear on the joints that robs them of their friction-reducing, cushioning layer of cartilage. At least 27 million adults are thought to have osteoarthritis. Another 1.3 million or more have rheumatoid arthritis.

These conditions can become expensive, as the authors of one *Archives of Internal Medicine* study noted in 2009. In 2005, nearly 500,000 total knee replacements—which are often used to treat arthritis—were performed at a cost of more than $11 billion. (That comes down to more than $20,000 per surgery.) This surgery is expected to become far more common in coming decades. People with osteoarthritis may see their annual out-of-pocket health costs increase by $694 (for men) to $1,379 (for women). In addition, having osteoarthritis increased the annual costs for patients' insurers by more than $4,000 for men and nearly $5,000 for women, according to an article in a 2009 issue of *Arthritis & Rheumatism.*

In terms of rheumatoid arthritis, another 2009 study from *Arthritis & Rheumatism* of more than 8,500 patients with the condition found that their average annual out-of-pocket expenses were $1,798. Forty-four percent of the patients said they had trouble paying their portion of the medical bills after insurance, and 9 percent had severe difficulty with bills.

Osteoarthritis becomes more likely as you get older, and rheumatoid arthritis is an autoimmune disorder that occurs when your body's immune system turns against your joints. However, neither condition is inevitable. You can take action to protect yourself from these conditions. Want evidence? Let's start by taking a look at Canada.

A 2010 study found that about 19 percent of Americans had arthritis compared to about 17 percent of Canadians. Americans were also more likely to have limitations on their daily activity from arthritis compared to their northern neighbors. The authors surmised that the difference was largely due to obesity and physical inactivity being more common in the United States. About 14 percent of Americans' arthritis burden is due to obesity, and 15 percent is due to physical activity.

It appears that you have at least some control over whether you'll someday naturally enjoy freedom from painful joints or whether you'll be paying a lot of money for treatments so your joints don't hurt as badly. Among the steps to take:

Keep your weight down. According to the Johns Hopkins Arthritis Center, obese women are nearly four times as likely to develop knee osteoarthritis, and obese men have nearly five times greater risk. Even being merely overweight has also been found to increase people's risk.

Protecting yourself from osteoarthritis by losing weight could save you major expenses down the road. You don't necessarily have to lose huge amounts of weight to protect yourself. If your BMI is higher than 25, even modest weight loss will help. **Be careful while being active.** Doing aerobic and strength-training activities that keep your legs strong and toned can help protect your joints. Regular physical activity is also important for keeping your weight at a healthy level.

However, injury to tissues in the knees will raise your risk of later osteoarthritis in that area. Use care when participating in sports and activities that could injure your knees. Warm up and cool down appropriately, gradually increase your intensity during activities (as opposed to diving in weekend-warrior style), always wear the proper footwear, and stay aware of your limitations.

Plenty of types of exercise are low or no impact, but help keep your joints moving, well lubricated, and healthy. It's been said that the only way to feed a joint is to move a joint. Consider swimming, water aerobics, stationary bicycling, walking, yoga, or tai chi.

Reduce your risk of rheumatoid arthritis. Some research suggests that you may be able to lower your risk of rheumatoid arthritis through your diet and other lifestyle choices.

One step that may be helpful is eating fish regularly. One 2009 study from Sweden found that people who ate oily fish one to seven times a week had a modestly lower risk of developing rheumatoid arthritis. Getting more vitamin D may also help lower your risk of the condition. Your body makes vitamin D if you expose your skin to a few minutes of sunlight daily (just a *few* minutes of unprotected sun exposure, though—see discussion in Chapter 4 on skin cancer), though the sunlight may not be strong enough in the winter if you live in northern latitudes. You can also get vitamin D from fortified low-fat or fat-free dairy foods and supplements.

In addition, you may also lower your risk of rheumatoid arthritis by not smoking. In a 2010 study from the *Annals of the Rheumatic Diseases,* researchers compiled the results of sixteen earlier studies and found that in men, current smokers were 87 percent more likely to have rheumatoid arthritis, and past smokers had a 76 percent higher risk. In women, current smokers were 31 percent more likely to have the condition, and past smokers were 22 percent more likely to have it.

Treating and Preventing
Ear Infection–Related Expenses

It's a situation that most parents—and *any* doctors who see children—have encountered at some point. Here's what it often looks like from the doctor's standpoint: The harried mom shows up midmorning with a red-faced, tear-streaked toddler who's tugging at her ear. Mom already knows what she wants from the doctor: antibiotics. After all, this ear infection is caused by bacteria, right? Just kill those germs with antibiotics and the child's pain goes away. The little girl feels better and will stop screaming. In addition, if she's been on antibiotics for twenty-four hours, her day care will let her return the next day.

So, doctor, how about those antibiotics now?

Ear infections provide a classic opportunity to approach a common problem with less intervention from a doctor. According to the American Academy of Pediatrics (AAP) and American Academy of Family Physicians (AAFP), American children develop more than 5 million cases of ear infections, also known as acute otitis media, each year. About 80 percent of these kids will get better *without* antibiotics. That bears repeating: **In most cases, your child doesn't need antibiotics for this problem.**

However, too many parents aren't giving their kids a chance to fight off the infection on their own. Half of all antibiotic prescriptions for preschoolers are written for ear infections. In 2000, roughly 80 percent of visits to the doctor's office in America for otitis media ended with an antibiotic.

This isn't good for your child, you, or your pocketbook. All this unnecessary use of antibiotics is giving ear infection–causing germs more chances to adapt to the drugs, making them ineffective in more and more cases. As a result, antibiotic-resistant cases of ear infection are becoming increasingly common. By seeking nonantibiotic solutions to your child's ear infections, you aren't just doing society a favor, you may be saving yourself—and your child—hundreds of dollars down the road.

Some evidence suggests that kids given antibiotics for ear infections are more likely to have more of them. A Dutch study from 2009 looked at 168 kids who were given either the antibiotic amoxicillin or a placebo—a substance with no medicinal value—for ear infections between the ages of six months and two years. Parents didn't know which one the child received. Over the next three years, 63 percent of kids receiving amoxicillin had recurrent ear infections, compared to 43 percent in the placebo group.

Still, perhaps an even bigger reason to avoid unnecessary antibiotics is the risk of drug resistance. Even a course or two of amoxicillin for ear infections can raise your child's risk of antibiotic resistance. If your child's ear infections become resistant to this relatively cheap drug, your doctor may need to move on to more expensive alternatives in the event that an antibiotic is necessary.

In addition, antibiotics can have unwanted side effects that you should avoid if possible. They cause nausea and vomiting in about 15 percent of kids—which are also common reasons for day care to send kids home. They can also cause allergic reactions in up to 5 percent of kids. You could end up incurring even more healthcare costs to treat these.

Here's some welcome news: after just twenty-four hours, the majority of kids will have improved symptoms, and up to 90 percent feel better within a few days, according to the AAP and the AAFP. The organizations point out that antibiotics *don't* relieve pain in the first twenty-four hours, and do little for pain after that. The groups released guidelines to doctors for treating ear infections, and they made a big push for doctors to use watchful waiting when appropriate. Simply watching the child for a while before giving antibiotics could save 3 million antibiotic prescriptions each year, they say.

According to the organizations, your doctor *should* use antibiotics:

- In infants under the age of six months if she suspects or is certain that the child has acute otitis media.
- In kids between six months and two years in certain cases or suspected cases with severe symptoms.
- In kids ages two to twelve years when the doctor is certain that your child has acute otitis media and the symptoms are severe.

These guidelines are only for healthy children, though—not kids who have had acute otitis media within thirty days or kids who have other serious conditions that could affect their ear infection, including a faulty immune system.

In cases where your doctor doesn't think antibiotics are needed, then watchful waiting is an option. Remember, watchful waiting isn't the same as no treatment. You're still keeping an eye on your child, and if the symptoms don't improve, *then* you can start the antibiotic prescription or other appropriate next step.

In the meantime, medication can help treat the symptom that's probably most upsetting—the pain. Pain relievers include acetaminophen (like you'll find in Children's Tylenol) and ibuprofen (such as in Motrin). Both of these are available over the counter. A cost-free source of pain relief is to put a warm pack—such as a washcloth dipped in warm water—against your child's ear.

During the infection, encourage your child to get plenty of rest. Rest is the body's built-in mechanism of restoration and healing. Providing plenty of fluids—water is best—is important, as the hydration helps thin secretions that can add to or cause painful pressure from congestion in the sinuses and ear canals. Avoiding milk may also be a good idea in times of acute infection, as dairy can increase secretions and worsen congestion.

In addition to avoiding dairy while in the acute phase, avoid decongestants, antihistamines, expectorants, and other over-the-counter cold remedies in treating an ear infection in your child. They won't provide much or any benefit, and may lead to side effects that make the situation worse, such as hyperactivity or trouble sleeping. In addition, experts now recommend against using many of these over-the-counter cold remedies in children younger than age four.

If at-home measures are not working, or your instinct says there is something more going on, honor that and call your doctor ASAP. If your child requires antibiotics, be sure to give them according to the label's directions. If you stop giving them when the symptoms ease, your child may still have lingering bacteria that can then develop resistance to the drug.

In addition to these treatment strategies, you may also be able to help prevent ear infections with these steps, most of which are completely free:

- Breast-feeding your infant for the first six months of life appears to help prevent ear infections early in life.
- Avoid putting your child to bed with a bottle; drinking from the bottle while lying down may contribute to infections.
- Limit pacifier use in babies and toddlers.
- Keep your child away from all tobacco smoke.

If your child's doctor recommends a follow-up visit, come in as scheduled. Even if your child seems well, there could be unresolved issues related to the ear infection that, left unattended, can lead to more time-consuming and costly health interventions down the road.

Preventing Infertility-Related Expenses

Although infertility doesn't pose a threat to your health in the same way that the other conditions in this chapter do, it can make a dramatic impact on your quality of life, your mental well-being, and your bank account. According to the CDC, in 2002 more than 7 million women had trouble conceiving or carrying a child to term, which was about 12 percent of women of reproductive age.

The uncertainty and frustration that can come with infertility can take an enormous emotional toll on women and their partners. So can the medical treatments to address infertility issues. Doctors can provide a range of treatments, including drugs and surgeries, depending on the specific problems that are interfering with conception or pregnancy. However, taking hormones, making trips to the doctor, and undergoing procedures can dramatically interfere with couples' home lives and work schedules.

The journey through treating infertility can also rank among the more expensive purchases a woman or couple will make in their lives. According to the American Society for Reproductive Medicine (ASRM), the average cost of an in vitro fertilization cycle is $12,400. This is a procedure in which eggs are retrieved from the woman and fertilized with sperm in the lab, then the resulting embryos are put back into the woman. A 2009 study in the *New England Journal of Medicine* found that among more than 6,100 women undergoing in vitro fertilization (IVF) in one facility, the rate of live birth after six cycles was between 51 and 72 percent, with rates substantially higher in women under thirty-five than in women forty or older. So couples may go through several cycles without success.

Health insurers often won't cover fertility treatments, so many women or couples have to pay for some or all of this medical care out of pocket. For some, the expense may be more than they can handle.

Although you can't always avoid infertility, in some cases women and men can take simple, inexpensive steps to prevent or treat its underlying causes. Even if you're not planning to start a family anytime soon, taking action now to protect your ability to conceive and carry a child could have a major impact on your quality of life and your finances in a few years.

Get PCOS under control. A condition called polycystic ovary syndrome (PCOS) affects between 5 and 10 percent of women of reproductive age (some experts suspect the percentage of women affected is actually much higher), and it's the most common cause of infertility in women.

If you're trying to get pregnant, PCOS can also be expensive. In a 2005 study, researchers estimated that the cost of treating infertility in women with PCOS in America was about $533 million in 2004. The authors also estimated that half of women with PCOS will seek infertility care during their lives, and the average cost per pregnancy is about $8,000.

Insulin resistance typically plays a role in PCOS, and up to 70 percent of women with PCOS are obese. But even women of normal weight can be affected—and this is an important point because normal body weight can throw a doctor off course in establishing the correct diagnosis. We have been taught that PCOS (similar to high cholesterol or high blood pressure) is only seen in reproductive-age patients with excess body weight—or in those with other telltale symptoms such as excessive hair growth, acne, or irregular periods. But this is simply not true—and a big reason why this condition is largely underdiagnosed.

Aside from the fertility risks, women with PCOS are also at higher risk of diabetes, cardiovascular disease, and problems during pregnancy, such as high blood pressure and gestational diabetes. In addition to the symptoms described above, there can be cysts on the ovaries, as well as certain hormonal abnormalities. But it is important to note here that all, some, or none of the symptoms can be present in a woman with PCOS. In some women with very mild PCOS with few to no outward symptoms, the only issue at hand may be the inability to achieve or maintain pregnancy due to impaired (rather than nonexistent) ovulation. In other words, the *quality* of the ovulation may be subpar, making a successful conception less likely.

Although you may need medications to treat certain aspects of PCOS, a healthful diet low in simple carbohydrates and sugar, regular physical activity, and shedding pounds if you're overweight go a long way toward dealing with the condition and its complications. According to the American College of Obstetricians and Gynecologists, daily exercise can help relieve symptoms of PCOS by improving the body's use of insulin. And weight loss alone may be enough to restore normal ovulation in some women. Weight loss has not only been linked to a greater chance of getting pregnant, but to improvements in excess body hair and blood sugar as well. The organization recommends that you lose weight by both cutting back on calories and getting at least thirty minutes of exercise daily.

Another low-cost method of treating PCOS and helping restore (or improve the quality of) ovulation is the prescription medication metformin. Generic versions are cheap, and some pharmacies may even offer it free with a prescription.

Protect your sexual and reproductive health. Sexually transmitted diseases can lead to later infertility and problems carrying a child full-term. A condition called pelvic inflammatory disease can result from the bacterial STDs gonorrhea and chlamydia. These bacteria can travel to a woman's uterus and fallopian tubes, leading to an unnoticed infection that can cause scar tissue, which can block these tubes. This can keep sperm from reaching the egg, or can cause a fertilized egg to grow larger in the tube or other location outside of the uterus, which is a serious condition called ectopic pregnancy.

About 10 percent of women with pelvic inflammatory disease become infertile, and the chances increase when women have it more than once, according to the CDC. As a woman's number of sex partners rises, her risk of pelvic inflammatory disease goes up as well. Having more than one partner at a time also raises her risk. Guys, take note: This risk goes for you, too. Chlamydia and gonorrhea infections can also scar the tubes that carry sperm out of the testes. Limiting your number of partners and using condoms can help lower your risk.

Another very common virus called human papillomavirus, or HPV, can also affect women's childbearing ability. HPV is very common in adults who are sexually active. According to the CDC, at least half of sexually active men and women will have it at some point in their lives. Usually, the virus doesn't cause health problems, and the body clears it away within a few years. However, some strains of HPV can cause genital warts and some cause cancers, such as cervical cancer. The virus can be passed from person to person during sexual activity. And according to the CDC, the virus can spread even if you're using condoms.

During regular checkups, a doctor may find worrisome changes in cells in a woman's cervix that are caused by HPV and may progress to cancer. These lesions may be surgically removed using different types of procedures. Removing these little spots of tissue may cause later problems during pregnancy. Depending on which procedure was used to remove the tissue, studies have found markedly higher risks of pregnancy complications, including severely premature delivery, low birth weight, and loss of the fetus, in women who have had cervical tissue removed.

Again, limiting the number of one's partners—whether you're a man or a woman—will reduce your overall risk of HPV. Girls and young women can also get protection from being vaccinated against strains of HPV that cause most cervical cancers. Boys may also be eligible for vaccination.

Preventing Injury-Related Expenses

In 2006, Americans made more than 27 million visits to emergency departments across the United States to be treated for accidental injuries, according to statistics from the CDC. They fell, were injured in car crashes, were hurt on bicycles, or got a foreign body stuck somewhere it didn't belong. Others were poisoned, burned, or got sick from overexertion in the hot sun.

People often think of "accidents" as something that transpires out of the blue sky and can't be avoided. Accidents *do* tend to come as a surprise when they happen, but in retrospect, they're often not surprising at all. In many cases, accidents can be prevented. While you're making tweaks in your life in order to stay out of the doctor's office or hospital, take steps to safeguard yourself and your loved ones from accidental injuries:

Be safe on the road. According to the National Highway Traffic Safety Administration, in 2004 the cost of not wearing seat belts in vehicles was $18 billion. Because people who aren't wearing seat belts during a crash tend to have more severe injuries, their costs of treatment are more than twice as high compared to people who are wearing a safety belt. The agency also points out that the average cost of inpatient rehabilitation for people injured in motor vehicle crashes is more than $11,000.

So, put on your seat belt every time you drive, even for short distances, and insist that your passengers do the same. Be sure that small children are riding in age-, height-, and weight-appropriate car seats or booster seats. Also remember that impairment starts with the first alcoholic beverage, and if you've been drinking, don't get into the driver's seat.

If you're hitting the road on two wheels instead of four, the Pedestrian and Bicycle Information Center recommends that bicyclists reduce their risk of injuries by:

- Always wearing a properly fitting helmet
- Riding *with* the traffic flow, not against it
- Staying off the cell phone and avoiding listening to music through headphones or earbuds while on the bike

🍲 Keeping a close eye on debris, storm grates, and slick spots on the road in front of you

🍲 Making sure you're visible if you're riding in the dark by having headlights, taillights, and reflectors on your bike, and wearing bright clothing

Be safe on the lawn. When you're mowing your lawn or cutting down weeds, be sure to wear shoes (not sandals) and protective eyewear. Don't let young children use lawnmowers or ride on riding mowers as a passenger. Pick up rocks, toys, sticks, and small objects when mowing so they don't fly out and hurt someone nearby. And as a matter of routine, just don't let your kids hang out close by when you are mowing . . . period. Use a mower with a safety device that stops the motor or the forward motion when you let go of the handle. And *never* reach under the mower to pull out an object when the blades are running.

Childproof and elder-proof your home. Kids and older people both have special needs when it comes to safety in the home. When childproofing your home to protect infants, toddlers, and small children, the U.S. Consumer Product Safety Commission recommends devices including:

🍲 Safety locks and latches for cabinets that contain household cleaners, knives, medicines, and other potentially harmful items

🍲 Safety gates to keep children away from stairs and out of rooms that may contain hazards

🍲 Smoke alarms on each level of the home

- Outlet covers for power outlets to help prevent electrocution
- Devices that keep the cords on window blinds from dangling within reach of small children
- Protective bumpers to cover sharp edges and corners of furniture and fireplaces
- Anchors for large furniture to help prevent crush injury
- Antiscald devices for faucets and showerheads to help prevent burns. Another tip is to turn the temperature down on your water heater to 120 degrees or less.

Older people should try to make their homes more easily navigated. A fall can result in broken bones and other serious injuries that can cause a loss of mobility and independence, and take a long time to heal. Ways to make homes safer for older people, according to the American Academy of Orthopaedic Surgeons, include:

- Installing handrails along stairs and grab bars near the toilet and along the tub
- Keeping stairways and walkways free of clutter and rugs that can slide
- Putting nonskid textured strips on the floor of the tub or shower
- Keeping a lamp and a telephone in an easily reachable spot near the bed
- Making sure phone and electric cords don't cross open areas of floor

Preventing Common Respiratory Infections

According to the National Institutes of Health, Americans have a *billion* colds each year. As a result, this is one of the more common reasons for doctor visits and missed school days. In addition, up to 20 percent of Americans have the flu each year.

Although colds may seem like a relatively minor hassle, both colds and flu leave a substantial financial impact on households. A 2003 study from the *Archives of Internal Medicine* found that nonflu viral respiratory tract infections (medical-speak for colds) cost nearly $40 billion each year in direct costs like over-the-counter drugs and treatment of complications like sinusitis and ear infections, and indirect costs related to days of missed school and work. A 2007 study from *Vaccine* found that annual flu outbreaks cost about $87 billion.

It's unlikely that you can totally avoid these infections, given that they're so common. However, if you can cut down on the number of colds and flu episodes that affect your household, you can certainly enjoy fewer missed days of work—due to your own sickness or your kids'—and cut down on complications from these illnesses, which can be serious and expensive.

Wash your hands. Regularly using a few cents' worth of soap and water may well be the most cost-effective way of keeping cold and flu viruses out of your system. According to the CDC, these illnesses are typically spread by germs that travel in droplets of moisture from coughs and sneezes. These may land directly on you from other people, or they may land on objects that you later touch and transfer to your own system.

The CDC recommends that you use soap and warm water to wash your hands for fifteen to twenty seconds or about the length of time it takes you to sing the song "Happy Birthday" twice. Wash your hands before you eat and after you sneeze, blow your nose, or cough. During cold and flu season, it doesn't hurt to wash them a little more often.

Be mindful of touching your face. Keep your hands away from your face. Your face offers several doorways into your body that germs love to enter: your nose, mouth, and eyes. Try to keep your hands and fingers away from these areas, especially during cold and flu season. If you simply must scratch, bite a fingernail, or attend to some other fingers-to-face task, wash your hands first. Getting mindful of how and when you touch your face is useful here as well. We'll get more into the concept of mindfulness in Chapter 7.

When I was in residency, I got engaged to my now husband. Our wedding was in November, which is a prime time for viral infections. Of course, as a doctor, I was exposed to illnesses nearly every day. So I was a little paranoid that I might get sick— perhaps with something visible such as pinkeye—for my wedding. A fellow resident had come down with ringworm before her wedding, on her face of all places, so this fueled my fire.

How could I protect myself when potential danger lurked behind every exam room door? I adopted the habit of never touching my face unless I was certain my hands were freshly washed. If I had an itch anywhere on my face and just had to address it right then, I grabbed a fresh tissue or paper towel and used that. I became mindful of touching/not touching my face, and it became a habit I maintain today. The result: My number of viral or other infectious illnesses went way down after that. And I got married healthy (with no ringworm in sight).

Use a tissue. Do a favor for bystanders who would like to cut their cold and flu costs, and use a disposable tissue to sneeze or blow your nose. Throw it away when you're done and wash your hands afterward. Encourage your kids and other housemates to follow these hygiene practices, too.

Avoid other people who are sick . . . Whenever possible, steer clear of people who are coughing, sneezing, blowing their nose, or showing other symptoms of illness.

. . . But get your shots, just in case. A vaccine against the cold isn't available, and probably won't be anytime soon (if ever). However, you can get a shot to lower your risk of the flu. The CDC now recommends that everyone six months and older get a flu shot each season, particularly those who are at high risk for complications or who are in close contact with someone at high risk. This includes: kids younger than five and adults sixty-five and older, pregnant women, and people with chronic conditions including asthma, chronic lung disease, and heart disease. Get your shot in the fall before the flu season peaks.

The CDC also recommends that certain groups get vaccinated for protection against pneumonia caused by *Streptococcus pneumoniae* bacteria. This pneumococcal polysaccharide vaccine is recommended for people sixty-five and older; younger people with chronic diseases such as heart disease, lung disease, and diabetes; smokers; and people with conditions that lower their resistance to infection, such as certain cancers and HIV infection.

Take care of yourself. By keeping yourself healthy, you may make your body more resistant to attacks from cold and flu viruses. Be sure to get plenty of sleep, eat a healthy diet, drink plenty of water, and try to limit your stress, particularly when the cold and flu are going around. And this is a good time for another plug for regular physical activity. A recent study published online in the *British Journal of Sports Medicine* found that people who exercised at least five days a week had 43 percent fewer days of upper respiratory tract symptoms than those who exercised one day a week or less.

Your New Prescription:

✓ Stay mindful of risks that face you—whether they're injuries around the home or illnesses that could be prevented with vaccination—and be proactive in taking steps to avoid them.

✓ Remember that even illnesses that seem minor can become costly hassles, such as the cold and flu. Free or inexpensive habits, from not touching your face to washing your hands more, can help prevent these common conditions.

✓ Keep in mind that one of the more upsetting and common conditions of childhood—an ear infection—doesn't necessarily require antibiotics.

✓ Keep eating sensibly and getting regular exercise. Being overweight doesn't just contribute to diseases that can kill you—it also puts you at risk of many problems that lower your quality of life.

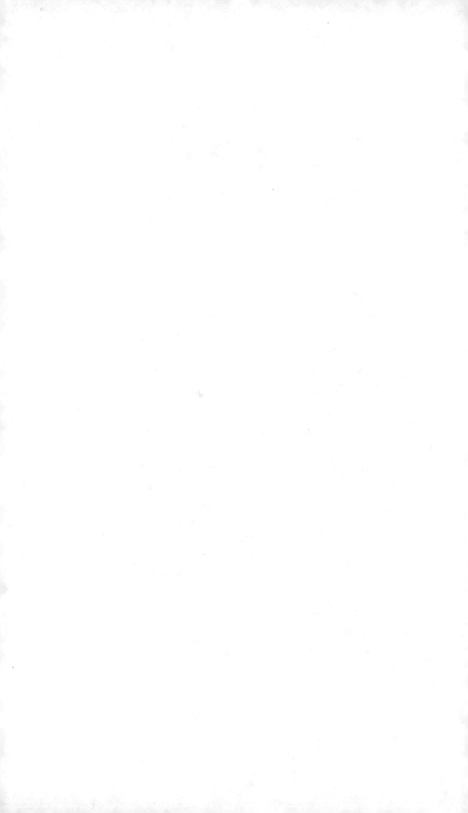

6

Treating Chronic Conditions Better, with Less Cost

It's a regular ritual we've seen many times: after the President receives his medical checkup, the American public learns the details about what the doctors discovered.

At one of these, President George W. Bush had a precancerous lesion on his arm treated, and his total cholesterol level was found to be a respectable 174. At an earlier checkup, President Clinton's total and "bad" LDL cholesterol were too high, but his rosacea (a skin condition) seemed well controlled, and his vocal cords were unchanged from earlier exams (an issue associated with gastrointestinal reflux disease [GERD] that was included due to his bouts of hoarseness). Interestingly, it was also noted in Clinton's health briefings that his GERD medication regimen was to be simplified "because after January 20th, he will be in charge of taking his own medications."

157

Nothing terribly exciting, but it gives the public something to talk about on a slow news day.

In the spring of 2010, some of the media coverage about President Obama's checkup took a slightly different tone. The good news was that the president was fit and trim, with a body mass index below 24. His resting pulse was low, and his blood pressure was at a healthy level. The not-so-good news was that his cholesterol was too high and that he still smoked.

But the *really* bad news to some people was that the president received unnecessary tests during his checkup. Rita Redberg, M.D., M.Sc., editor of the *Archives of Internal Medicine*, pointed out in an editorial that the president underwent an electron beam CT scan of his heart's arteries to look for coronary calcium. And he also underwent a "virtual colonoscopy," which uses another CT scan to create images of the colon to look for abnormal growths, without the need to insert a scope internally.

Both tests exposed the president to radiation, which carries a cancer risk. In addition, as the author pointed out, the president wouldn't fall within a risk category that warranted the coronary calcium scan, according to the U.S. Preventive Services Task Force (USPSTF), which issues recommendations for screening tests. And the USPSTF doesn't currently recommend using the virtual colonoscopy for screening due to insufficient evidence supporting it. Plus, these tests are expensive.

Quitting smoking for good would have helped his heart far more than knowing about whether calcium—found in plaques—was building up in his heart's arteries, the doctor pointed out, before she got to the real point:

"Some might defend these tests on the grounds that the President, of all people, deserves the very best our health care system can provide, but that would miss the point: more care is not necessarily better care," she wrote, adding that Obama's experience "is multiplied many times over at extraordinary cumulative financial cost to society and personal cost to the individuals who receive tests with known adverse effects and potential harms but without benefits."

So when the president receives what could be construed as the "executive physical" (a special physical exam designed for people who can pay out of pocket for any test they wish to have, despite some of these tests not falling in line with evidence-based medicine), what kind of message are we, as a society, getting? That more is better. Forget what the evidence says, forget what the guidelines of care say. Getting the newest, most cutting-edge *something* (or a lot of somethings) is the health care we want, the health care we need—if we could only afford it. But it's not (and none of us can afford to continue down this path, anyway).

So then, what *is* the health care we want, the health care we need? It's simple: We should seek *better* care—and only the health care we need. And it's simpler to get there than we as a society are making it.

We want to avoid the political finger-pointing that entangled the discussions of health reform. But we were elated to see that news outlets like NPR and *USA Today* also used President Obama's "first physical" as a teachable moment, just as we would have, if it had involved any prominent figure.

The point we're trying to make throughout this book is the one you just read: More care is not necessarily better care. The more expensive option isn't necessarily the better one. The more invasive procedure isn't necessarily the better one. The newest medication, device, or technique isn't necessarily the better one. Taking fast action isn't always better than taking a wait-and-see approach. In fact, these can all lead to worse outcomes in some cases. And though it may surprise you to hear this after decades of warnings that you should be screened for diseases such as cancer, sometimes even these screenings can be harmful. As it turns out, sometimes looking for problems isn't the best idea.

As you have learned in the previous chapters, you can save many thousands of dollars by preventing expensive, chronic diseases including diabetes, heart disease, cancer, and dementia, as well as more acute or self-limited illnesses such as colds and ear infections. But sometimes, despite our best efforts, we develop major or costly health problems anyway. When these medical issues arise, the choices you make can still have a big effect on how much your health care will cost. And instead of saving money years or decades from now, you can start tallying up savings now—while reaping major health gains along the way.

When Screenings Are a Smart Idea— and When They're Just Looking for Trouble

In March 2010, Richard Ablin, Ph.D., the discoverer of prostate-specific antigen, better known as PSA, wrote an opinion piece in the *New York Times* about the PSA test that's promoted as a way to catch prostate cancer early. He pointed out that about 30 million American men undergo PSA testing each year, at an annual cost of at least $3 billion. But Dr. Ablin wasn't writing to rejoice about the lifesaving effects of this test. Under the headline "The Great Prostate Mistake," he writes that the test's popularity is directly responsible for "a hugely expensive public health disaster."

While this test has helped save lives, the tide seems to be turning against the PSA, as experts run the numbers on the benefits and risks of the test. And the PSA is only one of the screenings that has gotten critical reappraisal in recent years.

In October 2009, the chief medical officer of the American Cancer Society, Otis Brawley, M.D., was quoted in the *New York Times* saying: "American medicine has overpromised when it comes to screening. The advantages to screening have been exaggerated."

Shortly afterward, the U.S. Preventive Services Task Force recommended that instead of starting routine annual mammograms at forty, women in their forties at average risk for breast cancer should discuss with their doctor when to start them, and from the age of fifty to seventy-four they should only have one every other year.

A few days later, the American College of Obstetricians and Gynecologists (ACOG) came out with new recommendations for Pap testing for cervical cancer that bumped back when women should start having them (at twenty-one, rather than three years after they become sexually active or at twenty-one, whichever was earlier), and spaced them further apart for some women (every other year for most women ages twenty-one to thirty, instead of every year, and once every three years for those age thirty and older who've had three consecutive normal tests).

These changes triggered a burst of outcries. The American Cancer Society voiced its support for continuing annual breast screenings for women at average risk in their forties. A former head of the National Institutes of Health said on a news program that "I'm saying very powerfully ignore them"—referring to the new guidelines for mammograms—"because unequivocally this will increase the number of women dying of breast cancer." The media carried stories of many women who found a serious breast cancer during screening. One online pundit wrote "HC (Health Care) Rationing Begins: Younger breast cancer victims not important enough."

It is indeed easy to point to women who are understandably vocal about the fact that they were screened in time to catch an early breast cancer. Our society focuses a lot of attention on pink ribbons, 5-kilometer (3.1-mile) runs for a cure, and the importance of being aware of breast cancer. How on earth could someone tell us to worry less about breast cancer? Why would women not check to see if they have breast cancer?

Because, as we're learning for several diseases, finding medical problems early doesn't necessarily mean we'll live longer, healthier lives. And for all the people you see whose lives were saved by a screening, you don't usually see the people who suffered through extreme anxiety over a test that told them incorrectly that they had a disease. And you don't see the people who underwent expensive, unnecessary biopsies and surgeries for suspected disease that turned out to be a false positive. You don't see the people undergoing additional surgeries, painful radiation, and chemotherapy for cancers or other diseases that may not have posed a serious threat to their health.

For example, in announcing its revised recommendations for cervical screening, the ACOG pointed out that human papillomavirus—the cause of most cervical cancers—is very common in sexually active adolescents. These young women tend to get many precancerous changes in their cervixes, too. But most of these lesions go away on their own without treatment, and invasive cervical cancer is rare in women under twenty-one, according to the ACOG. When you take into account that women may be more likely to give birth prematurely after having suspicious lesions cut out of their cervix, you may see a benefit in not tracking down and treating this group of women.

As another example, research now tells us that mammography may simply not be accurate enough in women under the age of forty, with high rates of false positives creating the need for additional imaging and procedures to result in an "all clear." Thus, the exposure to radiation may not tip the risk/benefit ratio to favor routine screening in younger women. It has also been reported in the medical literature that mammography has poorer screening outcomes in women forty to forty-nine years of age. Armed with all of this data, taking a second look at who stands to benefit from screening begins to look not so much like rationing, but rather more like appropriate (and higher-yielding) usage of radiation.

Let us be clear about our stance on screening here: Screening does save lives. And screening exams do play an important role in keeping you healthy. Catching a serious disease early in its process, which is the intention of screenings, can allow your doctors to treat the disease more effectively, more cost-efficiently, and with fewer interventions compared to catching it when it's further along.

However, sometimes catching a disease process early may mean stepping in and making major decisions when the threat—or the solution—isn't so clear-cut. As we already mentioned, an inappropriate screening test may lead to additional and more invasive procedures, which can then lead to physical and psychological suffering from the procedures themselves and possible adverse effects of any such procedure. And it can end up leading to wasted time, energy, money, and other resources—without leading to better outcomes.

Knowing when to use screenings can help ensure that you get their benefits without their costly drawbacks. Although we could detail the harms of excessive screening for breast cancer, cervical cancer, heart disease, and other diseases, a closer look at the PSA test for prostate cancer will offer some lessons we can apply to other parts of our health care.

A Screening Test Under Fire: PSA

The prostate is a small structure located beneath a man's bladder. In general, as long as it remains quiet, guys have little reason to give it much thought. Prostate-specific antigen, or PSA, is a type of protein that the gland produces. A number of conditions can make PSA rise in a man's bloodstream. PSA levels may go higher as the prostate grows larger, which is very common as men age, and levels may rise during inflammation of the prostate, which is also not uncommon. More serious, however, an increase in PSA can point to possible prostate cancer.

Prostate cancer is the most commonly diagnosed cancer in men, after skin cancer, accounting for about 218,000 cases in 2010. It's also the second most common cause of cancer-related death in men, killing an estimated 32,000 men in 2010. A number of celebrities have died of it (musician Frank Zappa, actors Dennis Hopper and Bill Bixby), and many are survivors (including Bob Dole, Robert DeNiro, Rudy Giuliani, and Colin Powell).

Two landmark studies in the early 1990s found a benefit of using PSA testing in combination with the more invasive digital rectal exam, in which the doctor feels the prostate through the rectum for abnormalities using a finger. Traditionally, a PSA lower than 4.0 ng/mL has been considered normal. As the number goes up, so does your risk of prostate cancer, in general. If it's between 4 and 10, you have about a 25 percent chance of having prostate cancer. If your PSA is higher than 10, you have more than a 50 percent chance.

So, what's not to like about an inexpensive, noninvasive blood test to catch this common cancer in its earliest stages? For starters, it's not a test for prostate cancer. It's a test for a lab value that can point to several problems, not all of them serious. In addition, although prostate cancer is very common in men, in many cases it may not pose a pressing health threat. And of special importance, treatments for prostate cancer may cause serious, unpleasant side effects—some of which can linger and cause torment for the rest of the man's life, quite drastically impacting his quality of that life.

Once a man finds out he has a high PSA, he may find himself sliding toward an expensive, life-changing surgery, and it can be really hard to get off this slippery slope once it's begun. In a 2008 study in the *Journal of Urology*, researchers checked for prostate cancer in 340 male organ donors who died suddenly of causes like strokes, car accidents, and trauma. Men in their sixties had a 33 percent chance of having prostate cancer, and men from ages seventy to eighty-one had a 46 percent chance. None of the men likely had any idea that they had the cancer. The PSA test may uncover many cases of prostate cancer that men otherwise would have gone their entire lives without knowing they had, until they died of something else.

For the cervix and colon, if screening finds growths that could progress to cancer, a doctor can oftentimes snip out the offending tissue relatively easily without a high risk of major side effects (although with regards to the cervix, these procedures may raise the risk of later pregnancy problems). But if men have their prostates removed through a radical prostatectomy, it has been estimated that about two-thirds could lose their erectile function and up to one-third have some degree of urinary incontinence. If radiation is used to treat the cancer, it may cause rectal damage, which can lead to problems with having bowel movements in some men.

In a study published in August 2009 in the *Journal of the National Cancer Institute*, researchers did some calculating and came to the conclusion that more than a million additional men had been diagnosed and treated for prostate cancer due to PSA screening—and most didn't benefit from finding the cancer early. Researchers chose to start looking at the year 1986, which was just before an important study pointed to PSA as a marker for prostate cancer, and just before the incidence of prostate cancer—in other words, newly diagnosed cases—leaped by an unprecedented number.

In 2005, compared to 1986, the incidence of prostate cancer in men under the age of fifty was more than seven times higher. In men in their fifties, the incidence was more than three times higher. Overall during this period, doctors found an estimated 1.3 million additional cases of prostate cancer than they would have found if PSA screening hadn't become available. And more than a million of these men were treated for the disease.

The authors estimated that during this time, approximately 56,500 prostate cancer deaths were prevented. If you knew you were one of those people, you'd most likely be happy with your investment in that PSA test. But what about the other men who were diagnosed and treated, but wouldn't have died from their cancer anyway? What did they get for their time, money, and trouble?

As the researchers pointed out, "Overdiagnosed patients cannot benefit from treatment because their disease is not destined to progress to cause symptoms or death . . . All over-diagnosed patients are needlessly exposed to the hassle factors of obtaining treatment, the financial implications of the diagnosis, and the anxieties associated with becoming a cancer patient—consequences that, by our estimate, have occurred among more than a million American men since the initiation of PSA screening."

Two other studies, reported earlier in 2009, also found more concerns for PSA screening. One study, with more than 162,000 men who either were or weren't offered PSA screening, found that PSA screening reduced the rate of death from prostate cancer by 20 percent, but 1,410 men would need to be screened to prevent one death from prostate cancer. The other study included nearly 77,000 men in America. The men were provided with annual screening or usual care (which often included screening). After seven years of follow-up, the study found no reduction in deaths from prostate cancer in men in the screening group. Outcomes at ten years were similar.

The first study also found that 75 percent of men who underwent a prostate biopsy to follow up on the PSA screening didn't have cancer. Thus, many of the men underwent an uncomfortable test—one that bears a risk of bleeding and infections—to find nothing.

It's true that cancer can escape the prostate and start growing elsewhere in the body. But it's also true that a slow-growing cancer can stay confined in your prostate for the rest of your life without ever causing a dire threat. Men who have had their prostate removed due to cancer might be inclined to say, "Well, at least I don't have that cancer in me anymore," even if the treatment cost thousands of dollars, required them to take time away from work, and left them with unpleasant side effects such as erectile dysfunction. But if you are aware of this possible outcome before you make the decision, would you choose differently?

More medical experts are starting to urge caution before men agree to PSA screening. Dr. Brawley, of the American Cancer Society, wrote an editorial to accompany the study that suggested more than a million men with prostate cancer had been overtreated.

As he pointed out, it's hard for doctors and laypeople to accept the idea that some cancers won't cause death, or even symptoms. Some treatments for prostate cancer "are very expensive and some have serious and long-lasting side effects. Little has been done to figure out which therapies are most effective. Every treatment looks good, when more than 90 percent of men getting it do not need it," he wrote, adding that "the irrational tendency to adopt treatments and technologies without adequate assessment is a form of 'medical gluttony' and a major reason that U.S. per capita healthcare costs are the highest in the world."

Howard Brody, M.D., Ph.D., director of the Institute for the Medical Humanities at the University of Texas Medical Branch in Galveston, told us that during his final ten years as a practicing physician, "I ended up having a lot of conversations with my male patients about the PSA. I'd start out by saying, 'If you want a PSA, I'm going to order it for you. No one's depriving you of a test. But before we order it, I want to be sure this is an informed decision on your part,'" he says. He would then tell them about the risk of harm versus benefit from the procedure, and many patients found this news "pretty dramatic."

Still, he points out, it's much easier for doctors to just do the PSA test on you and not have to worry that they could be sued later for not finding a case of prostate cancer if one arises. As a result, like we discussed in Chapter 2, it's important that screening discussions occur against a backdrop of a trusting doctor-patient relationship, where you're well informed of the benefits and risks of the test, and you're aware of the implications of your decision.

Is this the last say on the value of PSA screening? Not by a long shot. A study published in the summer of 2010 in the *Lancet Oncology* randomly assigned 20,000 middle-aged and older men to a group invited for PSA testing every two years or a group that wasn't invited. Over a fourteen-year period, prostate cancer mortality was reduced by almost half in the men in the screening group. However, the researchers found that "the risk of over-diagnosis is substantial," and 293 men needed to be invited for screening and 12 needed to be diagnosed to prevent one death from prostate cancer.

By no means should you take this as a blanket recommendation that men shouldn't have a PSA, or that men and women shouldn't have the variety of other screenings that are commonly recommended. These all have an important role in diagnosing and treating disease, and each screening test you encounter needs to be weighed according to its benefits and risks.

As another example, a 2010 study from the United Kingdom found that people who had a single flexible sigmoidoscopy—in which the doctor examines part of the colon—had a 33 percent lower chance of developing colorectal cancer in the next eleven years, and a 43 percent lower chance of dying of the disease. That's a pretty good benefit from one twenty-minute test.

This gets us back to the principle of having a primary care physician, and one with whom you feel comfortable, so that you can discuss your specific situation and the whys, hows, and what-fors of each screening's applicability to you.

In making sure you are getting the best health care in terms of screening, you need to ask questions before you proceed with any, and be aware that screening tests can lead—in some cases— to expensive and unnecessary treatment that brings additional risks. Keep the following suggestions in mind, no matter whether you're considering a screening for cancer, heart disease, or other conditions.

Talk to your doctor about whether a screening is truly appropriate for you, given your age, family history, and other risk factors. We've provided the latest screening recommendations from major medical organizations (see **"Check the Recommendations Before Screening"** on page

page 174). These can help guide you and your doctor's decision on screenings, but your individual factors also need to be weighed as well.

- Ask your doctor how sensitive and specific this test is (see **"Understand How Screening Tests Work"** on page page 173 for an explanation). Does this screening generate many false positives—an error that could cause you a lot of anxiety and needless follow-up treatment now—or a lot of false negatives, which is an error that could cause problems later?

- Remember that screenings aren't harmless. They can open the door to extremely costly medical treatments that may cause side effects, complications, and even death. In addition, the screenings themselves may cause injury, and those that use x-rays or CT scans expose you to radiation. Too many doctors and patients casually open this door without giving thought to what they'll do with the information they may find on the other side.

- Remember that a screening can come back with a false positive. How will you react to being told that you may have a disease? How well can you handle the anxiety that may ensue until further testing puts you in the clear? And will this information make any difference in your health outcomes?

Understand How Screening Tests Work

 Screening tests—whether they're looking for breast cancer, prostate cancer, or other conditions—don't necessarily provide clear-cut yes or no answers for whether or not
you have a condition or are at risk for it. Rather, they take
a measurement, then interpret whether your chemical level, x-ray
image, sample of cells, or other finding falls within what's considered "normal" or what suggests a problem.

Deciding what's normal and what's not is like fishing: You want
a net that's big enough—and with small enough holes—to grab the
fish you're seeking. If you use a small net with big holes, many of
the fish passing by will get away unnoticed. But use an enormous
net with tiny holes, and you'll grab up everything nearby, which
wastes your time and resources.

The *sensitivity* of a test is a measure of how many people who
really have the condition are identified by the test. In other words,
if 100 people really have precancerous growths in their colon, how
many will the screening test catch? The *specificity* of a test is a
measure of how many people out of a group that doesn't have a
problem are correctly identified as not having it. If 100 men have
a high number on their PSA test, how many actually have prostate
cancer and how many have benign causes of the elevation?

As a reminder, a false positive means the test identified you as
having a cause for concern that doesn't really exist. A false negative
means the test didn't identify a disease or a risk that you actually
have.

When a doctor recommends that you have a screening, ask if he
knows what the likelihood of a false positive or negative is before
you take the test. Remember that a false positive can cause a lot of
anxiety, and if it leads you to have further testing or treatment that
you don't really need, it can open the door to a lot of unnecessary
expense.

Check the Recommendations Before Screening

 Wondering whether a screening test is a good use of your money and time? Here are some recent guidelines from major organizations for who should have screenings and at what age. Keep in mind that these are general guidelines, and you and your doctor should also include your personal factors when making a decision. In addition, organizations vary on some guidelines. But the following recommendations should get you started.

Breast Cancer

U.S. Preventive Services Task Force (USPSTF), 2009: Women should have a screening mammography every other year between the ages of fifty and seventy-four. Any decision to start before fifty should take into account your beliefs regarding the benefits and harms of the screening. In women seventy-five and older, the evidence doesn't provide enough guidance on this test's benefits and harms.

American Cancer Society (ACS), as of 2010: Yearly mammograms starting at age forty and continuing while the woman is in good health.

Cervical Cancer

USPSTF, 2003: Women need cervical cancer screening if they've been sexually active and have a cervix. Women don't need routine screening if they're older than sixty-five, have had recent normal Pap smears, and aren't at high risk for the cancer. Women don't need routine Pap smear screening if they've had a total hysterectomy for benign disease (like fibroids).

ACS, as of 2010: Begin screening three years after beginning vaginal intercourse, but no later than age twenty-one. Do annually if using regular Pap or every other year using newer liquid-based Pap. At age thirty, women who have had three normal Pap tests in a row can be screened every two or three years. Women older than thirty also have the option of screening every three years with the conventional or liquid-based Pap plus the human papillomavirus (HPV) test. At the age of seventy, women who have had at least three normal Pap tests in a row, and no abnormal ones in the last ten years, may stop having them. Women who have had a total hysterectomy—which removes the cervix—for benign disease may stop the Pap tests.

American College of Obstetricians and Gynecologists, 2009: Begin screening at twenty-one, and do so every other year until the age of thirty, using standard Pap or liquid-based cytology. At thirty, those who have had three negative tests in a row may be screened every three years. Routine testing should be discontinued in women who have had a total hysterectomy for benign disease with no history of high-grade cervical intraepithelial neoplasia. ACOG also supports discontinuation of cervical cancer screening at age sixty-five or seventy among women with no abnormal results within ten years and three or more negative results in a row.

Colorectal Cancer

USPSTF, 2008: Adults ages fifty to seventy-five need screening using fecal occult blood testing, sigmoidoscopy, or colonoscopy. Guidelines recommend against routine screening of people ages seventy-six to eighty-five, with individual exceptions, and they recommend against screening people older than eighty-five. Evidence doesn't provide enough guidance on the benefits or harms of CT colonography and fecal DNA testing.

ACS, as of 2010: Beginning at age fifty (if at average risk), start having one of these: flexible sigmoidoscopy every five years; colonoscopy every ten years; double-contrast barium enema every five years; CT colonography every five years; annual fecal occult blood test; annual fecal immunochemical test; or stool DNA test. The first four tests are preferred when possible. People at higher than average risk should follow the screening schedule advised by their physician.

Prostate Cancer

USPSTF, 2008: Evidence is insufficient to weigh benefits and harms of prostate cancer screening in men younger than seventy-five, and the task force recommends against screening in men seventy-five and older.

ACS, as of 2010: Begin discussing pros and cons of screening at age fifty, or starting at age forty-five if you're African American or this cancer has affected your father or a brother before age sixty-five. Screening, if you opt for it, should include PSA with or without a digital rectal exam.

Coronary Heart Disease

USPSTF, 2004: The task force recommends against routinely screening people at low risk for coronary heart disease events with resting ECG, exercise treadmill test, or electron-beam CT to check for severe coronary artery narrowing or to predict coronary heart disease events. It couldn't find evidence for or against these screenings to assess the presence of severe coronary artery narrowing or to predict coronary heart disease events in adults at increased risk.

Osteoporosis

USPSTF, 2002: Women ages sixty-five and older should be routinely screened for osteoporosis. This should begin at sixty for women with higher risk of osteoporotic fractures. It makes no recommendation for or against routine screening in postmenopausal women younger than sixty or women from sixty to sixty-four without higher risk of osteoporotic fractures.

Abdominal Aortic Aneurysm

USPSTF, 2005: Men ages sixty-five to seventy-five who have ever smoked should have a onetime screening. The organization makes no recommendation for or against screening in men of this age who have never smoked, and it recommends against routine screening in women.

Look Both Ways Before Leaping into a Big Procedure

In the summer of 2009, physician and *New Yorker* writer Atul Gawande, who often writes about problems facing our health-care system and their potential solutions, penned a story that made a splash.

In it, he traveled to McAllen, Texas, where healthcare spending per person is nearly the highest in the nation. Medicare spends $7,000 more per person in this city than it does in the average American city, but the care there doesn't appear better, he writes.

In his story, a surgeon described a trend of surgeons removing patients' gallbladders instead of advising the patients to change their diets, offering pain medication, and perhaps keeping an eye on gallbladder flare-ups to see if they would go away on their own. The author pointed to evidence suggesting that patients in the town got more testing, more surgeries and other treatments, and "more of pretty much everything" compared to the national average.

This serves as a good reminder that if a thousand patients with the same condition walked into doctors' offices or hospitals around the country on the same day, they wouldn't all get the single "right" treatment. Some may be more likely to receive surgery. Some might be more likely to be treated with medication. Some doctors would want to work fast and aggressively with their patients. Other doctors may propose a "watchful waiting" approach. This means in many cases, if you develop a serious or chronic condition, you and your doctor may be able to work together in planning an approach that can treat you more effectively and more cost-effectively—or in essence, *better*.

One organization that's been calling attention for years to differences in healthcare services across our country is the Dartmouth Institute for Health Policy & Clinical Practice. In its 2008 Dartmouth Atlas of Health Care, the authors point out that the rate at which doctors admit patients with chronic diseases to the hospital is very much related to the number of hospital beds per person in that area. And the number of visits made to specialists is related to the number of specialists in the area.

In addition, the authors point out, people with chronic illnesses don't have better survival or quality of life if they live in an area with more medical care available. In fact, their outcomes may be worse. One explanation is that every time you're tested or treated, there's another opportunity for something to go wrong. Spending time in the hospital puts you at risk for picking up infections from nasty germs that lurk there. More testing creates more opportunities to find issues that wouldn't have bothered you if you'd never found them, which the authors call "pseudodisease." Surgeries and other procedures that are powerful enough to help you are also powerful enough to harm you.

"Regions of the country and hospitals with low rates of utilization are not rationing valuable care: quite the opposite. Rather, regions and hospitals with high rates of utilization may in fact be overtreating patients. They are delivering unnecessary care, which is not producing better outcomes," the authors write. You can apply this to your own life, as well. Using fewer and more carefully focused health services for your medical problems doesn't necessarily mean you're not getting what you need. It may just mean you're not getting what you don't really want.

Douglas Wood, M.D., a cardiologist and the chair of the division of healthcare policy and research at the Mayo Clinic, is familiar with the idea that major procedures aren't always done because they're the best solution for the patient. In McAllen, Texas, which has a sky-high rate of bypass surgery for blocked coronary arteries, some of the patients having these surgeries may have traveled south for the winter from places like Dr. Wood's area in Minnesota, he says. "Our surgical rate is very low. Had they been here in the winter, they probably wouldn't have gotten their bypass operations."

In coming years, the medical profession may be taking a more critical look at whether patients need the vast numbers of expensive surgeries they're currently getting. It's in your best interest to be ready. You will already know what you really need and what you really want, which is how to get better care at a more afford-able price—and enjoy better health.

In a January 2010 issue of the *New England Journal of Medicine*, Howard Brody, M.D., penned a commentary calling for each medical specialty to come up with a "top five" list of diagnostic tests or treatments that are often ordered, especially expensive, and shown by evidence to not be particularly beneficial to many patients who receive them. Though it should be easy enough to find general agreement about the five best candidates, some spe-cialties could even have a top twenty or fifty list, he told us. Each specialty then should teach its physicians to discourage the use of these procedures in patients not likely to get benefit from them.

He says he's gotten good feedback from the medical commu-nity for his stance. "E-mail has been overwhelmingly positive. A few physicians get angry and say, 'How dare you imply that I'm ripping off my patients?' But so many people have responded positively. They used words like courage and bravery, though I didn't see it that way at all."

Dr. Wood relayed a story of a patient he'd seen recently, which illustrates the availability of many different solutions for most problems. The man was in his fifties—a prime time for heart dis-ease in men—and he'd had CT imaging to look for calcification in his coronary arteries, which (as mentioned in our President Obama example) points to a buildup of plaque in the arteries. Though the man had no symptoms, his cardiologist told him that he did have some plaque. Further, the plaque's location in an especially important artery was a "widowmaker problem" and that if it led to a heart attack, it would be fatal. As a result, the patient was told he quickly needed a catheterization, which is an invasive procedure that would enable a good view of his coronary arteries and an opportunity to open up narrowed areas if necessary.

"He actually hesitated and said, 'I'd like a different opinion about this,'" Dr. Wood told us. "He came to Mayo, we did a stress test, and he did extremely well. I said, 'You don't need a heart catheterization. You need to work on minimizing your risk for a heart attack.' He spent money for our consultation and a couple of other tests, but it was a lot less expensive than spending $20,000 for a heart catheterization and angioplasty."

While impossible to say for sure, one could also argue that he received not only more cost-effective health care, he received better health care. And he definitely headed off the potential risks of a catheterization at the pass.

Just as certain areas of the country appear to spend unnecessarily high amounts on health care, so do individuals and families. And they can take steps to change their spending habits immediately.

"There is just as big a difference between two families with the same conditions who live right next to each other in McAllen or El Paso as there is between the two towns," says Don Kemper, M.P.H., the founder of Healthwise, an Idaho-based company that focuses on empowering patients to make more well-informed decisions. "It's how people respond to their illness, and how they participate in their decisions, and what they're willing to do for themselves that can have an even bigger difference than the geographic variance in the way their doctors practice. Patient responsibility, careful shared decision making, and looking for the most cost-effective and responsible actions can reduce our healthcare costs in half."

If you've developed a serious condition and a doctor recommends an expensive procedure to treat it, it's wise for you to put some time into researching your options before you sign on the dotted line. If you're having a medical emergency and require immediate treatment, the following advice may not apply. But if you have the time to weigh your options, consider these steps:

Ask the doctor if you really need to have the treatment. Dr. Wood says, "If you're going to your heart specialist and he says 'Your stress test is abnormal, you ought to have a heart catheterization,' and you're not having many symptoms, you have to ask, 'Do I really need this?'"

Ask why the doctor has recommended this course of action. Does evidence support that this treatment is better than the less-expensive or less-invasive alternatives? Does research suggest that you're the kind of patient who will get the most value from this procedure? What kind of long-term outcomes do patients have from this procedure in terms of survival, freedom from disability, and quality of life?

Ask what other options are available. "If you have coronary artery disease," Dr. Wood says, "we know now that your outcome over ten years will be the same if you start with medications as your treatment, if you start with angioplasty and a stent, or if you start out with bypass surgery. We've learned that for people with few or minimal symptoms with their coronary disease, they don't need anything more than really aggressive treatment of their underlying risk factors. They don't need lots of imaging, they don't need catheterizations, they don't need angioplasty, and they don't need surgery."

In other words, quitting smoking can do a lot more for your heart health than a CT scan of your coronary arteries. It's better, more responsible health care and *you* hold all the power.

Ask whether you can improve your health on your own. On the topic of personal health empowerment, there are many tips toward self-reliance we want you to know. Although medications may cost less over the short term than a surgery that can cost five figures, medications may be excessively expensive and not a bit helpful if you don't really need them, or if you can avoid them by doing some work on your own. For example, if your doctor wants to put you on medications to control your blood pressure or diabetes, you could be on these for decades (if you rely on them to do all the work for you). Instead, ask if losing weight, improving your diet, and getting more exercise could help you avoid or delay needing these medications, or allow you to take less of them.

Ask whether "watchful waiting" may be a way to go. Researchers are finding that an approach called "watchful waiting," also known as "active surveillance," is an appropriate choice for some men with prostate cancer. Experts are appreciating the wisdom of considering watchful waiting instead of always rushing in with treatments for other conditions, too (like holding off on antibiotics for ear infections). With prostate cancer, for example, doctors can assess whether the tumor appears aggressive and life-threatening, or if it may remain quietly within the prostate without harming your health.

Active surveillance doesn't mean you're not doing anything. It means you're not using major interventions yet while your doctor periodically checks to make sure things aren't getting worse. If you're on active surveillance for prostate cancer, for example, future tests that show that the tumor is growing or showing ominous signs may suggest that you need to stop watching and start treating it.

Keep in mind that watchful waiting isn't necessarily an easy choice. You have to have a mind-set that allows you to go on enjoying your life even though you may still have a disease that's ongoing.

Get a second opinion. Consider talking to another specialist to gather more insight on the possible ways to approach your case, Dr. Wood suggests. Or bring your test results back to your primary care provider and discuss your specialist's recommendations. Specialists can become accustomed to providing the procedures they do regularly. Having a different perspective on the matter (along with less financial stake in the outcome of your decision, it should be said), your primary care doctor may be able to suggest different ways of approaching the problem.

Be a well-informed decision maker. Experts these days are talking more about concepts called "shared decision making" and "informed decision making," as Kemper mentioned earlier. These approaches may help you make more cost-effective choices concerning medical treatments. They may also lead to medical treatments that more closely fit your needs and lead to better outcomes.

Come to the table armed with knowledge about your options, the end results you would like to see, and an understanding of the risks you're willing to accept from the procedure. In addition to gathering advice from your doctors, this requires you to do research on your own so you can fully share in this decision.

After all, you're the one who will be responsible for going through the treatment, paying for it, and dealing with its consequences, not your doctors. Since this is such an important issue, in the next section you'll learn how to ask more questions and come up with the facts that will help you make better-informed decisions.

✦ ✦ ✦

Be Well Informed

"I used to have to go to people and beg them, and now they won't leave me alone," laughs Kate Clay, M.A., R.N., the program director of the Center for Shared Decision Making at the Dartmouth-Hitchcock Medical Center in Lebanon, New Hampshire. In the eight years she's been helping patients make health choices based on their values, she's seen interest in informed decision making grow substantially.

For patients faced with options for their health problems, the center provides decision aids on DVD, online, and in booklets, as well as in-person counseling. The materials are different from traditional patient education handouts. These help patients figure out which possible risks and benefits are most important and how the possible outcomes of their options line up with their values, Clay says.

Some of the center's thirty videos—produced by the Foundation for Informed Medical Decision Making in collaboration with Health Dialog, Inc.—are for so-called "preference-sensitive" conditions, where there is more than one reasonable choice, which should be driven by the patient's values and life circumstances. These are conditions in which the decisions should come down to the patient, such as people considering elective knee replacement for osteoarthritis, and they're cases in which having surgery affects the quality rather than the length of their life. Decision aids cover a range of topics, such as early-stage breast cancer, herniated discs in the back, weight loss surgery, PSA and other screenings, uterine fibroids, and how to address chronic conditions like diabetes.

Kemper, whose nonprofit organization also produces patient decision aids, notes that, "The good patient is no longer someone who goes and listens to the doctor and does what he says. The good patient today is informed and participates in her care.

"For every major treatment decision, testing decision, or drug decision, you want to go through a patient decision aid to help you determine if—all things weighed in the process—this is the right treatment for you now. Making those kinds of decisions can have a huge impact on your pocketbook," he says. "Cardiac care is a big area where the incentives are so in place to do open-heart surgeries, stents, and other very expensive procedures, even when the evidence is not clear that it would help a particular patient. Patients need evidence so they can make a judgment based on their condition and preferences, and then decide if these very expensive and invasive procedures are appropriate for them."

Too often, Clay says, a patient may "go to the knee surgeon and they say 'You have knee osteoarthritis. We could put you right onto the schedule for surgery.' The patient should be saying 'What are my alternatives here? Let me think about if I'm ready for this or if I'd rather get physical therapy, take medications, and lose weight.' And the physician should be saying, 'Let's talk about this and see what you want to do.'" She recalls talking to an acquaintance about her recent knee replacement for osteoarthritis. The surgery occurred after a conversation in which the surgeon told her friend, "You have bone rubbing against bone, and you need to have that replaced." Clay remarks, "He scared her with that 'bone on bone' comment. He never asked her if that option worked for her. If he'd asked her that, she wouldn't have had that surgery."

I have my own experience with deciding whether or not a major, potentially life-changing surgery was the right solution to a health problem. When I was around the age of twelve, I was diagnosed with scoliosis, a condition in which the spine begins to

curve abnormally. It never caused any problems during adoles-
cence, thus we never took any drastic steps to treat it. However,
I would eventually wear a brace and try various exercises and
physical therapies while practicing watchful waiting.

Still, in my twenties, I began shrinking in height, which wasn't
a good sign. The condition eventually progressed severely, and it
was going to keep getting worse—with the potential for heart and
lung damage and a shortened life expectancy. I was a newlywed
in my late twenties with my career just getting off the ground. My
husband and I very much wanted to start our family, so I needed
to take action and figure this thing out. I got a second opinion on
what my best course of action was, and the clear solution was to
proceed with a major back surgery to halt the rapid progression
of the curvature.

Now when I write "major back surgery," it really takes me
back. It is a funny thing, the doctor becoming the patient. I knew
about this kind of surgery because I studied it in school (and
avoided it during surgical rounds).

So I was somewhat prepared. But I also instinctively knew
that, while I needed my surgical team to do the surgery and
related procedures, a lot of the outcome was really up to me.
Rather than this feeling like a burden or frightening me, I felt
empowered. There were things I could do that would improve
my chances of the best surgical outcome, the quickest path to
recovery, and the lowest risk of complications.

Before the surgery, I lined up a support network to get me ready
for the surgery and help get me through my recuperation. This

included talking with former patients of my surgeon, who offered me valuable tips and information that helped calm my nerves. It also included rallying the troops of my immediate family, making sure I had "support staff" on hand to help me as I healed.

I also made sure I was eating well, getting adequate amounts of good quality sleep, exercising regularly, and getting into the right frame of mind for surgery and the rehabilitation that lay ahead. Being physically fit has always been a part of my life, but this was really the first time I started to see fitness as a tool in the armamentarium for fighting back to wellness. So I was ready, and I did it: I had the surgery, started the rehab, healed pretty darn quickly, and walked out of the hospital on my thirtieth birthday—two inches taller than when I went in.

At home, the recovery continued. And it wasn't easy. But I followed all the instructions that were given to me, which included walking early and often. It did not escape me that walking was an integral part of the healing process—it tends to help the bones fuse (fusion is a big part of the scoliosis surgery process). Within three weeks, I was completely off all pain medications and within six weeks, I was back at work full-time. And I should add that I gave birth to my first child within eighteen months after the surgery.

My back is now fused nearly from top to bottom with numerous rods that will remain for the rest of my life. I went on to have another child, and I continue to exercise regularly and live a very physically active life. This includes the regular mastery of a variety of new yoga poses, I am proud to report.

I give my surgeon and the rest of the surgical team the lion's share of the credit for doing a great job with the procedure (thanks for not messin' me up, Doc!), but I also know that I had a lot to do with it, too. *You* have a lot to do with your health outcomes as well—much more than perhaps you previously realized.

It starts with being as well informed as possible. And this is a three-parter. You not only need to get educated on your health matters, you then need to communicate well on your health matters. Third, you have to properly implement what you've learned and what you have communicated and what has, in turn, been communicated to you.

It's about getting the best care you can. And in the process, it's likely going to save you money. Clay says that the patients she works with don't tell her that they're learning how to make well-informed health decisions in order to save money. In fact, although some evidence suggests that when patients understand their values and the risks and benefits of their options they tend to choose less-invasive treatments, research has found that being informed could make people more likely to choose a surgery in some cases, because they are choosing what is right for them once they are well informed, she says.

However, setting aside whether or not being more well informed will save you money in every instance, we still think that it's the necessary approach, whichever kind of treatment you're considering. After all, you're going to be investing different types of resources in your treatment: money, possibly time away from work, help from loved ones and friends to take you on trips to the doctor or hospital, and recuperation time. Aside from the financial cost, you'll want to make sure that you're getting the most return on this investment of your resources. Being fully informed will help you do this.

When you're choosing between options for a major health concern, ask your doctor if he or she can point you toward patient decision-aid materials designed for your condition. If your doctor or hospital doesn't have them, your employer or health insurer may be able to provide them (that is, if you're not self-employed or uninsured). If you're facing a decision for a problem for which you can't find a decision aid, Clay suggests a form called the Ottawa Personal Decision Guide from the Ottawa Hospital Research Institute that helps you compile answers to relevant questions on one page. You can find it at http://decisionaid.ohri.ca/decguide.html.

If you're going to make a major health-related decision without the help of a decision aid, Clay offers four questions to ask yourself while weighing your options:

Are you well informed? Do you have solid information, based on good evidence, to support your decision? Good evidence comes from places like major studies in peer-reviewed medical journals, as opposed to a consumer magazine or a chat group you found online, she says.

Are you applying your values to this decision? "Do a little self-examination and ask yourself, 'What matters to me the most here?'" Clay says. All decisions carry a trade-off between risks and benefits. Attach some importance to each of these factors so you can decide which risks you want to avoid the most, or which benefits you most hope to gain.

Do you have sufficient support? Will family, friends, and other important people in your life help make your choice a success? Do the people whose opinions you value the most support your decision?

Are you sure about your decision? If you still sense some unease or have any hesitation, perhaps you need a second opinion from another doctor or more information to answer an important question that still lingers.

In addition, getting back to the knee-surgery example, Kemper advises that you include what you hope to do with your knees. If you love to play tennis, perhaps one option will be better. If you love to ski, perhaps another option will be more suitable. If you simply want to preserve your ability to walk around and live independently, perhaps another option is best. For any surgery or procedure, keep in mind the kind of lifestyle you'll want to live afterward—and whether the procedure will help you do it.

Follow Doctor's Orders

If the most expensive medical treatment you can buy is the treatment you didn't really need, then this kind of treatment may be the second-most expensive: the treatment that you and your doctor decided that you need, which you've already paid for, and that you're not using.

This is a major concern in medicine these days. One word for it is "noncompliance," which means not doing what the doctor suggests. However, the word "compliance" implies that the doctor's role is to give orders and the patient's role is to follow them, like a teacher and student or parent and child. So the word that's being used more often now is "nonadherence," which means the patient isn't sticking to the agreed-upon plan. Nonadherence runs up a lot of medical costs in America. Research has found that nonadherence to medications fuels about $100 billion in added costs each year.

Although Americans filled nearly 4 billion prescriptions in 2008 that cost $234 billion, many of those pills, tablets, injections, and liquids didn't get into people's bodies where they could do what was intended. Researchers have found that patients with chronic diseases typically only take half of their prescribed doses. Nearly a quarter of people take less than the label recommends. Twelve percent of patients don't fill their prescription at all. Another 12 percent don't take any of the medication after they buy the prescription. Former surgeon general C. Everett Koop said it well when he said, "Drugs don't work in people who don't take them."

When you have a chronic condition, not sticking to the plan of attack can run up your healthcare costs in many ways. If your condition gets worse because you're not keeping it in check with medication, the complications could require bigger, more expensive interventions. You may need to make more visits to the doctor's office. Your doctor may need to spend more time revising your disease-control strategy. And your doctor may not be as interested in working with you on shared medical decisions that save you money if you're not showing that you're interested in adhering to the existing plan.

In one 2005 study that followed more than 137,000 people with diabetes, high blood pressure, high cholesterol, or heart failure, better medication adherence was associated with lower hospitalization rates. In addition, in people with diabetes, for example, those with the best medication adherence had about $7,600 lower healthcare costs, even though they had higher medication costs.

People have a lot of reasons for not sticking with a medication regimen. They start feeling better and don't feel as compelled to keep taking the drug; they get tired of taking multiple drugs each day; they're taking the drugs to prevent a problem that seems like a distant threat (nonadherence is a particular problem for blood pressure medications, for example); they're having bothersome side effects; they don't feel like the drugs are helping; or they're having trouble paying for the drugs. Of course, people also can be nonadherent to other treatments besides medications, such as healthy lifestyle changes that could help keep a health problem in check.

Following our approach may help you better adhere to your doctor's plan for addressing your health problems. And keep these suggestions in mind when discussing medications or other long-term treatments that will require your participation:

Ask the usual questions. Before you agree to drug therapy, ask your doctor if the medication is truly necessary and proven to work for your condition. Are other options available that you would find preferable?

For example, prescriptions for proton pump inhibitors—used for reducing stomach acid—are filled more than 113 million times each year in America. However, researchers have found that these drugs are overprescribed, and at least half of these prescriptions are for inappropriate conditions. An editorial in a May 2010 issue of the *Archives of Internal Medicine* pointed out that these drugs have been associated with a higher risk of fractures in older women, a higher risk of pneumonia, and a higher risk of *Clostridium difficile* infection, which affects the colon and can lead to issues including diarrhea, sepsis, and even death. If you knew that a "harmless" stomach acid drug wasn't always so harmless, would lifestyle modification (such as cutting out acid-producing foods, quitting smoking, cutting back on alcohol, and losing a few pounds) sound more appealing?

Taking this approach with any remedy your doctor suggests might be well worth your while. Would losing weight, getting more physical activity, or taking any other steps provide the same benefit as this medication—without side effects? If a medication is in fact necessary, is a less-expensive version available?

If you do go with the medication, ask about benefits and side effects. If it causes side effects, is there anything you can do to prevent or alleviate them? What benefit is the medication supposed to provide? If the benefits will be noticeable to you, how long before you start to see them? If you're bothered by the side effects or aren't noticing a benefit, when should you call the doctor?

If you become nonadherent, ask yourself why. People who stop taking their drugs may not put a lot of thought into why they're quitting or what they could do to stick with them. Hopefully you have a clear understanding of why you need the treatment, and you trust your doctor's approach because you have a good relationship and you made the decision together. Instead of just stopping the drug, investigate the reasons why you're having trouble taking it, and see if you can find a solution.

Discuss your concerns with your pharmacist, or make a follow-up visit to your doctor, and try to find solutions instead of just giving up.

Get a Professional on Your Side

In some cases, having an advocate to help research the best treatments or healthcare providers or to escort you through an often complicated medical system may help you get more effective health care—and possibly save you money, says Laura Weil, director of the master's program in health advocacy at Sarah Lawrence College in Bronxville, New York.

"Let's say you have a new diagnosis of congestive heart failure. This is something you'll live with the rest of your life. Good management of the disease will help you live longer, stay out of the hospital, and save money in the long run," she says. Just having someone to help you understand and act on the discharge instructions when you're released from the hospital after a major procedure or serious health problem could make a difference in your outcome, she says, since patients often don't follow these instructions because harried hospital staff may communicate them poorly and anxious patients frequently don't adequately understand them.

Patient advocates may have a background in nursing or health care, and some may have a specific degree in health advocacy. On the other hand, the field is unregulated and some people with no particular training are calling themselves health advocates, Weil says. If you decide to hire an advocate, take some time beforehand to find out this person's background and qualifications. Make sure the advocate has experience working with your particular age-group and has plenty of experience with your particular health need. Also check to make sure the candidate is the best choice for the task with which you need assistance, whether it's dealing with your insurer or going on doctor's visits with you. Understand how much the advocate charges, and how many hours will likely be required to address your needs.

And be sure to look for advocates who may already be available to you. Your employer may provide access to a patient advocate as a benefit. In addition, Weil points out, many hospitals offer patient advocates as a free service. You may find them listed under patient representatives or as employees in the patient relations department. If you're having a problem while in the hospital, such as difficulty finding an answer or getting what you need from a physician, the in-house advocate may be able to arrange a solution. In these cases, an insider is likely to have better access to fix your problem than someone you bring in on your own from the outside.

Reduce the Risk of Medical Errors

An often-quoted 1999 report from the Institute of Medicine estimated that preventable medical errors in hospitals cost $17 to $29 billion each year in the United States. The organization defined medical errors as "the failure of a planned action to be completed as intended or the use of a wrong plan to achieve an aim."

These include serious errors like surgeons operating on the wrong body part or providers giving a massive dose of medication due to a math error. But plenty of errors occur in the healthcare setting that are more subtle. One example is that patients are at risk of developing infections that would have been preventable with a little extra care on the part of the provider, such as hospital nurses not washing their hands after each patient encounter.

Although in some cases the provider is responsible for treating the consequences of the error at no charge to you, oftentimes the patients or their insurers have to pick up the costs of additional treatment to address the error. Although you can't guarantee that an error won't occur when you go into the hospital or doctor's office, you can make these incidents less likely. Here's some advice from the Agency for Healthcare Research and Quality:

- If you have any choice in selecting a hospital for a procedure, choose one that does a high volume of your type of case. Outcomes tend to be better in hospitals with more experience with a specific procedure.

- Gently ask all providers to wash their hands before they touch you. This may be embarrassing to do, but it can really cut your risk of developing an infection, and infections you pick up in the healthcare setting can be quite bad. There's no telling what is lurking on surfaces that your doctor or nurse has recently touched. Healthcare providers know they need to wash their hands frequently, but it's a chore that can fall by the wayside in the bustle of a day. Don't assume and don't be shy. If your provider does not wash his hands in your presence, speak up and ask that he do so.

- Periodically have your doctor review all your medications, herbs, and supplements during a doctor visit. This can help reduce your risk of harmful interactions.

- Fully understand how to use a medication when your doctor prescribes it. Know when to take it, what side effects to watch out for, and whether you need to use any special precautions while taking it.

- When you pick up a medication at the pharmacy, ask for verification that it's the correct medication and dosage that your doctor prescribed.

- If you're going in for surgery, ask what you can do to ensure that the proper body part will be targeted. For example, if the surgery is on your left knee, ask the doctor or nurse to initial the proper knee with a pen or marker—or ask if you can do it yourself. It may seem funny that you'd have to say, "You know which leg you are operating on, right?" But it is not so funny if you wake up to it having been done wrong—and it does happen.

In addition, stay involved in your care. This has been the central message of this entire book for getting better care and better guarding your bank account, and it's particularly important for guarding your health (and your money) from medical errors. If you're in the hospital, try to pay attention to who's coming in and out of your room and what they're doing. As best as you can, know which medications you're taking, what they look like, and how often you should be taking them. If you have friends or loved ones helping you in the hospital, ask them to keep an eye on things, too.

One more (potentially controversial) tip: If you're planning an elective surgery at a teaching hospital, consider scheduling it for some other month than July. This is when fresh medical graduates begin their residencies and start caring for patients. Although this topic is in need of more research, in one study published in May 2010 in the *Journal of General Internal Medicine*, researchers found that dating back to the late 1970s, fatal medication errors in medical institutions jump by 10 percent in July in counties with teaching hospitals. The more teaching hospitals in an area, the bigger the spike.

Your New Prescription:

✓ Screenings play a valuable role in detecting diseases early in their process, and they can save lives. But they are not always necessary. When you do undergo screenings, you should do so with the knowledge that they may lead to worrisome news, false positives, and unnecessary care. Investigate whether you fall within a general group that should get benefit from a screening, and discuss with your healthcare provider whether your individual risk factors make a screening a good idea.

✓ If a doctor recommends a major procedure or surgery—and it's not clearly an emergency—invest the time to investigate your options. Get a second opinion. Is a more conservative approach a possibility? Can you do anything on your own to alleviate the condition and avoid the need for the procedure?

✓ Go into major health decisions fully informed. Understand your options and try to anticipate how these options will mesh with your values. What results do you hope to get from a surgical procedure? What risks are you willing to tolerate? Do you have sufficient support from the people around you to help make your choice a success?

✓ Stick with the plan you and your doctor devised. If you need to be on a medication, take it properly. If the two of you have decided that you need to change your lifestyle to reduce your health risk, do it. As you might have suspected by now, good health doesn't magically arise from spending fifteen minutes with your doctor. It comes from the work you put into it between appointments. Strive to follow the course of action.

✓ If you're facing a complex course of medical treatments and you feel like you're in over your head, consider hiring an advocate. Just be sure to research the advocate's qualifications, be clear about what you hope to accomplish, and understand the advocate's potential costs and benefits.

7

Developing the
New Prescription Mind-Set

Your doctors had to absorb a massive amount of knowledge before they could become qualified to treat medical conditions or help you avoid them. They took years of chemistry and biology just to get into medical school, where they spent another four years memorizing and absorbing bookshelves of information.

After more sleepless years of residencies, visits with hundreds or thousands of patients, and regular continuing education, your doctors have reformatted and reprogrammed their brains to deliver medicine. When they walk into the exam room with you, they're mentally equipped to investigate and help solve your problems.

But *you're* a crucial player in your health, too. As you've seen throughout this book, making choices that allow you to use more carefully focused healthcare services—while saving you time, energy, and money in the process—takes a lot of knowledge and insight on your part. If you're not well informed and well equipped, you're less likely to accomplish your health goals.

As you've moved through the chapters in this book, you've been adding new skills to your mental toolbox. You've learned how to make the best use of a doctor visit. You've learned how just a handful of behaviors, when practiced day to day, will help you stay healthy with less need for costly healthcare services. You've learned how to compile key information into a checklist to make better-informed medical decisions that suit your needs.

All of these are valuable skills. But to truly get into a healthier, wealthier, and wiser frame of mind, you'll want to bolster your knowledge base and adjust your perspective in other ways, too. For starters, it's important to develop a mind-set that allows you to monitor your health without becoming so concerned about it that you use unnecessary health care to address fleeting symptoms and minor problems. You'll also want to become a savvy consumer of the health information that surrounds us twenty-four hours a day. And you may need to bolster your ability to change your health-related behaviors once and for all.

The Costs of Too Much Health Anxiety

Protecting our health requires us to pay a certain amount of attention to our bodies' warning signals. Odd lumps that hang around, lingering coughs, unusual pains, worrisome moles, and unexpected bleeding will likely require evaluation from your healthcare provider. Acting quickly when the situation demands it can help head off health problems early in the process when a less-expensive and easier treatment may fix them.

On the other hand, focusing too much attention and concern on your health can run up your healthcare costs unnecessarily. For example, excessive worry can spur you to visit the doctor for passing symptoms and minor problems that would have gone away on their own. In addition, stress and depression can lead to many bothersome symptoms such as headaches and muscle aches. Acknowledging and addressing the emotional issues rather than just the physical symptoms can lead to better outcomes. As a result, recognizing the role of mental factors in your physical health is important for developing a cost-effective mind-set.

Jonathan Abramowitz, Ph.D., director of the Anxiety & Stress Disorders Clinic at the University of North Carolina in Chapel Hill and the author of *Treatment of Health Anxiety and Hypochondriasis*, often works with people who have a type of "health anxiety." Another term for this particular problem—which has picked up negative connotations over time—is *hypochondriasis*.

Health anxiety can affect people in severe or mild ways. In more extreme cases, says Dr. Abramowitz, health anxiety has led people to uproot their lives and move closer to prestigious hospitals because they're determined that only a world-renowned doctor can diagnose and treat their disease. Anxiety over their health may spur people to inspect each stool carefully for blood or test the acidity of their urine every time with litmus paper. Or they may spend hours online looking up their symptoms or calling doctor after doctor to discuss their concerns. Dr. Abramowitz has known of people driven to these extremes even when they had no physical problems that a doctor could detect. (And I can attest that even doctors can fall prey to health anxiety, too.) Many people may not act in such extreme ways, yet may still be bothered by health-related anxiety. "The interesting thing is, as soon as you get concerned about your health, a whole bunch of new symptoms seem to appear," he notes.

Physicians—especially primary care providers—often deal with an issue known as *medically unexplained symptoms.* A more medical term for this is *somatization.* These are aches, pains, twitches, fatigue, and other symptoms that the patient feels, but that aren't arising from any kind of physical disease process that the doctor can diagnose. Researchers have estimated that approximately one-half or more of all people seeing doctors in an outpatient setting have little to no physical disease that explains their symptoms.

Having medically unexplained symptoms can lead to a number of financial and health implications. Patients with medically unexplained symptoms may "doctor-hop," bouncing from doctor to doctor without establishing a meaningful connection with any of them. Doctors can find it difficult and frustrating to work with patients with these issues, which isn't the basis for a good doctor-patient relationship.

Other research has found that patients with somatization tend to take more sick leave from work and are more likely to report restricted activity. A 2005 study in the *Archives of General Psychiatry* of more than 1,500 patients—299 of whom appeared to have somatization—found that these people made more visits to primary care providers, specialists, and emergency departments, and had more hospital admissions. The annual cost of medical care for the somatizing patients was $2,734 higher than for other patients. As a result, the authors estimated that $256 *billion* a year in healthcare costs may be due to somatization.

Aside from the cost, symptoms that aren't due to an underlying physical problem can lead people to have unnecessary tests, medical treatments, and surgical procedures that can cause harm without the hope of a benefit to help balance it out.

As Dr. Abramowitz points out, not all symptoms require any particular treatment: in many cases, it's just "body noise," like a little background static from a radio. "We tell patients that everyone has a noisy body," he says. He reminds patients that we're willing to accept a little static from the radio without thinking that something's wrong with it. That's just how radios work. For that matter, when our computers freeze up or act a little odd from time to time, most of us just reboot the device and don't further investigate the problem—as opposed to disassembling the machine or taking it to the computer repair shop every time it acts up.

Dr. Abramowitz's approach to patients with health anxiety is to help them change the thoughts and behaviors related to their health. Here's how you can prevent health anxiety or better cope with it:

Change your focus. "People with health anxiety focus on the *possibility* rather than the *probability*," he says. As we discussed earlier in the book, when you come to the doctor with symptoms, she'll run through a list of so-called differential diagnoses. The list of possible causes of a hoarse voice and sore throat could include acid refluxing up from the stomach, a cold or other viral infection, or possibly throat cancer. Yes, all are possibilities, and if you visit a website that offers an online check-your-symptoms quiz, it will probably tell you all of them. But your odds of this symptom having a more run-of-the-mill cause are much greater than something dire like cancer. All kinds of other symptoms are much more likely to have a trivial explanation—or no observable explanation at all—than a terrible underlying disease. So, try not to jump to the worst possible explanation for your symptoms when a more benign diagnosis is more likely.

Recognize incorrect assumptions. Health anxiety can compel people to worry that "if I don't get to the doctor immediately, if I wait one more second, there won't be anyone who can help me," says Dr. Abramowitz. Some issues *are* medical emergencies that demand a quick trip to the doctor or a call to 911, such as strokes, heart attacks, poisonings, severe bleeding, and other traumas. It's important to keep some perspective on which problems are truly important, and which are likely to be minor issues or merely passing symptoms.

Stop pestering yourself. It's common for people to be concerned about their health from time to time. Health anxiety becomes a problem when it interferes with your daily life or causes you distress, Dr. Abramowitz says. If it has reached a point where it's a problem in your life, discuss it with your doctor or a mental health provider.

In my experience, I see patients sometimes on a regular basis solely as a therapy for their health anxiety. We're both aware that they don't have a physical problem that I need to diagnose or treat, but they feel they must see me on a regular basis until we get them past their anxiety. And it works.

Another option is to try to just stop the behaviors associated with your anxiety, Dr. Abramowitz recommends. If your doctor has told you that you don't have a particular disease—and you've developed a good relationship that should allow you to trust the doctor—then stop going to more doctors and asking for more tests (unless new symptoms arise or your symptoms become more severe). If you know what your doctor is going to say when you discuss a problem you've already addressed, ask yourself if you really need to be scheduling another visit. Avoid going to "diagnose my symptoms" websites over and over. Put an end to inspecting the body part or feeling a bump that your doctor has already cleared. Try to let it go and write it off as "body noise."

A special note applies here: actively listen to that inner voice of intuition; if you still feel strongly that there is something wrong, a second opinion (bringing along all previous test results, of course) is generally a good idea, especially if you're concerned that this is a potentially life-threatening issue.

Acknowledge the possible role of mental and emotional factors. People don't generally like to be told "it's all in your head," and they may think of that phrase if their doctor suggests that depression, anxiety, or other nonphysical issues could be playing a role in physical symptoms.

If you have a physical symptom that's bothering you, then you deserve to be evaluated by your healthcare provider for potential physical causes. But be willing to discuss what else is going on in your life that may be playing a role. Your mind and body are interconnected, and what affects one can affect the other. If your doctor suspects depression or anxiety, then mention whether you're having job or family stress, a death in the family, trouble sleeping, or other issues that can affect your mood or emotions.

And know that depression and anxiety can strike even when everything is going along swimmingly. This can be a major reason why people feel resistant to these problems as a factor in physical symptoms. They may think, "What do I have to be depressed or anxious about?" Many times, these afflictions arise simply due to chemical changes in the brain and have nothing at all to do with life circumstances. Still, more often than not, there are lifestyle issues—such as not getting adequate sleep, as one example—that do play a role. Addressing these problems or treating emotional issues with counseling or medications may help with the physical symptoms and improve overall well-being.

Practice Mindfulness

Both authors of this book are fans of the concept called "mindfulness." This means becoming more aware of where you are and how you feel in the present moment. It means instead of dwelling on your worries, try to set them aside and refocus on the here and now. It means taking inventory on a regular basis of how your body is feeling *right now*. When troublesome thoughts repeatedly intrude into your mind, don't argue with them or reason with them or worry about them. You acknowledge them, allow them to flow out of your mind, and refocus on the real world that's in front of you at the moment. As my father, a philosophizing family doctor and active practitioner and teacher of meditation, likes to say, "Suffering comes from dwelling on the past and worrying about the future. And neither is real. All that we have that is real is the here and now."

Sounds good, right? But how do you implement it? A simple tool in bringing things back to the here and now is this: When you find yourself suffering, ask yourself, "Am I dwelling on the past or worrying about the future?" Probably so. Sit quietly, start to check in with yourself—mentally scanning your body and releasing tension—and repeat to yourself silently, "All that is, is here and now. And right at this moment, all is as it should be."

Can this help you get better health in a broken system? Emphatically, yes. First, being more mindful may be a useful tool in addressing depression and anxiety—including anxiety about your health. Practicing mindfulness can also lead to reduced stress and stress hormone levels, in turn leading to reduced risk of a veritable potpourri of chronic, stress-related health ills, including heart disease, diabetes, and even cancer.

And, arguably most important, mindfulness can help give you a more accurate reading of the signals that your body is sending you, such as signs and symptoms that you truly have an issue that requires medical attention, or conversely that you're probably okay. In other words, "Patient, know thyself," and you'll be well on your way to getting what you need from the healthcare system, more efficiently and more cost-effectively.

Be a Savvy Consumer of Health Information

Since you've decided to pick up and read this book, you likely have reasonable reading skills. But how is your health literacy? Many people don't have the ability to understand and navigate the often-complex health information surrounding us as well as they could.

Health literacy, according to the federal government's Healthy People 2010 plan for improving our nation's health, is: "The degree to which individuals have the capacity to obtain, process, and understand basic health information and services needed to make appropriate health decisions."

Health literacy can be related to your ability to read—but it encompasses a lot more, says Christina Zarcadoolas, Ph.D., a health literacy expert at the Mount Sinai School of Medicine in New York City. "The biggest mistake is people say, 'Literacy—isn't that reading, writing, and doing math?' Well, no. Health literacy isn't just about understanding the language of health. It's understanding concepts, understanding the role of prevention, understanding complex issues, and then making decisions and changing behaviors based on good information."

You need a certain ability to understand health information in order to assess whether materials you find online are from a reputable or sketchy source. You need certain skills to understand the dosage on a medication bottle. You need to know what basic medical terminology means. For example, in terms of cancer, "negative" is good news and "positive" is more ominous, despite how they sound. You need to know why you should take a full prescription for your antibiotic, and which health risks are most important to you at a particular age.

According to the National Network of Libraries of Medicine (NN/LM), health literacy involves being able to seek out information and analyze it, decipher graphs and tables, and understand numbers. People who may be more likely to have limited health literacy skills include those who didn't graduate from high school or go to college, older people with cognitive problems, and people with chronic physical or mental conditions.

According to an Institute of Medicine report from 2004, about 90 million American adults "have difficulty understanding and acting upon health information." That's a considerable chunk of the population. Poor health literacy is costly in terms of money and lost health. A 2007 report estimated that low health literacy costs the U.S. economy between $106 and $238 billion each year. Low or inadequate health literacy has been associated with more hospital visits, improper use of medications, less use of preventive care, poorer health outcomes, and higher mortality rates.

Even with the popularity of health-related books, magazines, and websites, many people aren't savvy enough consumers of all this health information, Dr. Zarcadoolas says. "We're over-fed and undernourished when it comes to health information. Clearly, over the last fifty years, what we've seen is that pumping up the volume and putting more information out there per se hasn't created a more engaged, more health-literate consumer."

We can't tell you exactly how to assess the gaps in your health literacy and fix them; after all, as Dr. Zarcadoolas points out, you only find out how much or little you know about cars when yours breaks down. And you're unlikely to educate yourself about automotive mechanics ahead of time so you're ready for a breakdown. But here are a few ways to help ensure that you're getting accurate health-related information and understanding it correctly:

Go to reliable sources. If you need to learn more about a particular condition, a good starting point is with the websites from reputable associations that focus on the disease, such as the American Cancer Society, the American Heart Association, and the American Diabetes Association.

The federal government's National Institutes of Health and Centers for Disease Control and Prevention also offer a great deal of reliable information. Many of their documents are geared toward people with limited literacy skills, and they often provide animated movies that help explain complex topics.

Ask your doctor for more information. Your doctor likely has pamphlets and educational materials available for a variety of conditions. Hospitals, particularly large ones, may have patient education departments that can also provide useful materials. At your doctor's visit, ask if any educational materials are available. Be sure to specify if you'd like materials that are especially easy to understand, or ask him to go through it with you if you find you still have questions.

Take notes and speak up. For many reasons, a doctor's office might not be the best place to absorb new information, Dr. Zarcadoolas says. It's an unfamiliar environment, the doctor has a limited amount of time, and you may be upset about news you've just learned. As a result, many people leave the doctor's office without fully understanding the information they're given. This is not uncommon. Know that many people are in the same boat.

You have several options for capturing what the doctor tells you. Consider bringing a tape recorder or digital recorder and turn it on—with your doctor's permission—when he's sharing his recommendations. Or take notes in a notebook. Or bring along a friend or family member who can help you remember.

When the doctor tells you the medication regimen you should take or other steps you should follow, repeat it back to him to make sure you understand. If you have any questions at all or something still seems fuzzy, now is the time to ask the doctor for clarification. You can also ask your pharmacist for more clarification when you pick up the prescription.

Research published in August 2010 in the *Archives of Internal Medicine* found that the medication information that accompanied two types of drugs from 365 pharmacies was often difficult to use. Often these leaflets were difficult to follow and were written at an advanced reading level, and in some cases were extremely lengthy. These materials can be useful to consult, but your pharmacist is there to help too. Know that if you have questions or have been given information but are struggling to understand it, many other people probably feel exactly the same way. Don't be too shy or embarrassed to speak up and get the information you need. Ask your pharmacist to fully explain anything you don't feel comfortable with.

If you get home and find that you still have questions, call the office back and ask to speak with the doctor or the doctor's nurse or other staff assistant. If you *still* don't receive the information you seek, stay with it until you do. If you continually feel unable to get the answers you want, it may be time to look for a new provider.

Look deeper. When you're checking out health information online, pay attention to who's responsible for the information or paying for it. Is it a pharmaceutical company? An organization with a particular ax to grind? Someone selling a particular treatment? Does the source have something to gain—possibly at your expense? Keep in mind that economic and other factors may be influencing their point of view.

Also, when you're looking at websites, check out when the information was last updated. Was it checked for timeliness in the past year or two, or not since 1997? Medical knowledge is constantly evolving, and materials more than a few years old may be outdated. Was it reviewed by an outside medical expert? Many sites will tell you if they had another pair of eyes looking at the information, which helps ensure accuracy. But, again, this does not trump the date. Outdated material in the world of medical communications is simply not good enough to rely on in matters of your health.

Be critical of what you read in the news. Take some time before you revamp your treatment approach—or get worked up with anxiety—over health-related information you've seen in the media. Newspapers, magazines, and websites typically focus on the new and novel, like cool high-tech treatments and scary health threats. However, they may not have the space or interest to talk about the less exciting details, like side effects of a new treatment or the actual risk that individuals will develop a disease. Or how a new, expensive medication stacks up cost/benefit-wise against a boring old generic that's been around for years. They often don't put breaking news into a larger context, explaining how it fits into the big picture.

For example, a 2010 study in the *Archives of Internal Medicine* looked at 436 articles related to cancer that were published in national magazines and large newspapers. More focused on survival rather than death and dying, only a few (13 percent) discussed the possibility that aggressive treatments can fail, and only 30 percent mentioned that aggressive treatments can lead to adverse events.

In short, pay attention and stay well informed about health news, but remember that no news story offers the entire story—or the last word—on a health-related issue. And once again, always consider the sources. What do they stand to gain, if anything?

For a lot of mainstream media, it is about more attention (also known as "more eyeballs"). What better way to get that than through sensational headlines! Plain old facts and sensible advice tend not to sell as well.

Finally Change Your Health Behaviors

As you saw in Chapters 4 and 5, which showed you how to protect yourself from potentially life-changing and costly conditions, a small number of steps stand to offer big benefits. These steps are inexpensive or free, and they're extremely easy to remember. The most important ones are to eat nutritious foods in limited amounts, get regular physical activity, keep your weight down, and don't smoke. Stay with us . . .

Here's the problem: **Most people have heard this advice many times.**

It's quite possible that just the phrase "healthy living" makes you want to nod off. And most of us know that we should do these things. But the notion of reducing the risk of illness later simply isn't compelling enough to motivate many people to change their behaviors or make sacrifices now. We made a point of telling you exactly what kind of expenses you can sidestep by preventing diabetes, heart disease, cancer, arthritis, and other conditions. We suspect that these are facts that might be new to many people. Still, this information may slip your mind the next time you eye a pint of ice cream or reach for a pack of cigarettes.

After all, one chocolate chip cookie isn't going to make a substantial difference in your weight or your health. In addition, people who change their behaviors now to be healthier have to pay some kind of price: exercising more or quitting smoking involves effort, sacrifice, and maybe even inconvenience and discomfort.

A steady stream of your choices over a long period will make an impact. Those momentary costs you're paying now in terms of time, sweat, and a few more vegetables and a few less cookies can save you from big financial costs later. As you're developing a cost-cutting mind-set, an issue of prime importance is how to finally develop new behaviors that will support good health in the long run.

The recommendations on how to eat better, lose weight, and quit smoking could fill entire bookshelves. But you can get started on *all* of these improvements by following a few simple steps, says Leslie Martin, Ph.D., a professor of psychology at La Sierra University in Riverside, California, and coauthor of *Health Behavior Change and Treatment Adherence.*

Know why you want to change. Sure, we all want to be healthy in the future. But that's kind of an abstract notion that may not motivate your daily decisions. Why do you want to be healthy? Sit down and write out specific reasons why you want to be free of diabetes, obesity, or heart disease. Perhaps you want to look better and feel more energetic. Or you want to be able to enjoy your retirement after a long career. Or you want to be around to see your grandkids grow up, unlike family members who died of preventable diseases when you were young. These specific desires may give you some extra motivation.

As for me, I intend to be fully mobile, cognitively intact, and vibrant well into my nineties, just like my beloved maternal grandmother, who left this world following a stroke that came while she tended her tomatoes at the age of ninety-three. I know that it takes work to get there. But it's work that is well worth the effort. My Nonnie? She was of hearty German stock, yes. But she supplemented this generously with a very physically active life (going out dancing was one of her favorite activities, even into her eighties and beyond, and gardening . . . and those tomatoes—oh! those tomatoes—she tended them all, every year). In addition, she enjoyed a long and happy marriage to my (also very beloved) Bompo, a robust social network, and a smoke-free existence, and she placed *profound* importance on home-cooked meals (fast food was not on her menu, and I am pretty sure she didn't ever even hear the term "partially hydrogenated"). But I sure can recall her chicken . . . I digress.

So that's my simple goal. Live on like Nonnie did: in great health until the end. To get there, I have my own personal road map, and it's really about making each day count. Making each decision count. It all adds up to get you where you want—and need—to be.

Once you have some specific goals, write down your specific behaviors that are either helping or hindering your ability to reach these targets, Dr. Martin suggests. "It can be helpful to see written down the conflict or disparity between your present behavior and what you want in the future," she says. Are you still sneaking a few cigarettes here and there? Do items from your company's vending machine account for a sizable percentage of your daily calories? Are you getting too little sleep? Are these factors going to help you in your journey through a life that's less burdened with costly illnesses? It may also help to make your goals public—share them with someone or several people. This can help keep you accountable.

Figure out where you are in your readiness. An idea that's popular among experts who try to improve people's health behaviors is called "stages of change." It acknowledges that out of a group of people, some will be more willing to start changing a behavior than others.

Some people aren't planning to take any action in the next six months, but some are thinking about making a change in the near future. Others have come up with a plan of action and they hope to start in the next month, and yet others have already taken action and they're trying to avoid a relapse. Others have been maintaining their changes over a long period and they're not as apt to resume their old habits.

People at different stages need different motivations, Dr. Martin says, and you need to stick with actions that suit your current stage—not someone else's. "Doing something tailored for a more advanced change will set you up for failure," she says. For example, if you're hardly interested in improving your diet, suddenly throwing out all your desserts and high-fat foods is unlikely to lead to long-term success.

However, if you're not interested in making any changes in the near future, ask yourself why. What's holding you back? How could you develop a plan of action that would be appealing enough that you would want to get started? As you do start thinking about making changes, plan ahead and assemble your resources ahead of time instead of making a big change at the spur of the moment. Know what you're going to do, how you're going to reward your successes, and how you'll get back on track if you have a relapse. Line up friends and family to support your changes before you begin.

If you've decided to quit smoking, the American Cancer Society suggests that you decide on a quit day in the near future. In the meantime, you should get all your ducks in a row before the day arrives. Talk to your doctor about medications that can help, write down your reasons for why you want to quit, and line up support and encouragement. I also suggest to my patients to start physically and mentally preparing themselves and their environment well before the day of change arrives. In the case of quitting smoking, this means you will want to begin to erase the presence of tobacco well before your quit date. Get rid of ashtrays, lighters, matches, and other smoking accoutrements in your home and workplace, clean out your car, and take your clothing to the dry cleaner. Start to identify yourself as a *non-*smoker. Getting yourself into a frame of mind that smoking is no longer convenient, no longer a part of your routine, and no longer *wanted* goes a long way.

The same holds true for making changes in your diet and exercise routine. Starting to phase out old, unhealthy patterns and making way for new, healthier ones will help you transition more gracefully, and this leads to better sustainability, which is where the true benefits lie. Some tips here include cleaning out your pantry and eliminating foods that will trigger overeating or a downward slide. If you feel like you simply don't have any time to exercise at all during the day, try setting your alarm just thirty minutes earlier and ease into getting up and doing fifteen to thirty minutes of floor exercises before you get ready for the rest of your day, then move on from there.

Tackling smaller goals. It all starts with one step. If your boss simply told you at your annual review to "do better in the coming year," how helpful would you find that goal? How would you know where to set your sights? How would you know when you accomplished it? Similarly, "Don't get heart disease" is not a very specific goal for developing good health behaviors. Nor is "lose weight" or "eat better."

Instead, break these down into small, manageable goals that you can tackle in a shorter period so you can see quicker results. Aim for a ten-pound weight loss instead. Decide that you'll eat another serving of fresh fruits and vegetables each day next week. The following week, eat two more servings each day, until you're eating five to nine servings daily. Sign up to walk a 5-kilometer (3.1-mile) run/walk in your community, and start training for it. If you enjoy it, sign up for another one and make plans to shave a minute off your time.

These goals are right in front of you and they feel good when you attain them. If you can string a steady flow of these minigoals together over the years, you'll be frequently rewarded while you stay healthier. And you won't have to live your life with ponderously big goals looming in front of you. Remember what my father says: all that is real is here and now. This works for us here, too. If you think that you have to exercise and eat perfectly every day for the rest of your life, you are setting yourself up for misery. It's not about the future. It's about today: the here and now. Today you can choose to make healthier decisions. And if you choose a less healthy choice, that's okay too. Enjoy it and let it go. When that moment is gone, it becomes the past. Every moment is a new moment in which you can make a different choice, choosing to go healthier this next time around.

Stick with things you like. Many people *like* to eat French fries. They *like* to smoke. They *like* to watch sporting events on TV more than actually playing them. As a result, it's tough to make yourself switch a behavior that you like for one that you don't like, Dr. Martin points out. So instead of forcing a new unpleasant behavior on yourself, seek out choices that you actually enjoy.

If you actually enjoy bran and Brussels sprouts, by all means put them on your dinner table. But if you don't, find something you like better. If you like Thai food, get a Thai cookbook and experiment with delicious new vegetables and low-fat sauces. Try different types of exercises until you find ones you enjoy. If you don't like to run, then don't make it the centerpiece of your exercise regimen. Rotate between several activities that appeal to you so you don't get bored doing the same thing. If you're giving up smoking, find something else that provides relaxation and plea-sure to help replace the enjoyment that you get from cigarettes.

Whatever you do, make sure that your healthy new life is fun. Crash diets and short-term extreme changes aren't the foun-dation of a healthy life. You need to follow healthy habits for decades, not just a few months, and few people willingly stick with habits that they don't enjoy for long.

But one more thing here: keep in mind that many of those things you think you like, you probably really don't. You're a smoker? Think back to the first time you picked one up and took a drag. Probably wasn't too fun, was it? It was likely for other reasons that you kept doing it: peer pressure, looking for a release, something new to while away the time, perhaps? But you learned to like it, essentially teaching your body how much it needs this thing, and now you're hooked. Can't live without it. Same goes for regular soda or nightly ice cream. You can just fall into a habit that isn't good for you by repetition—training your body into craving what it then thinks it needs. The great news is that this also holds true for healthy habits.

Have you ever noticed how when you are on track with regu-lar workouts, when you miss a day you kind of miss the workout? Use this to your advantage. Start to build your routines around healthier behaviors that, over time, your body will begin to crave. It may take some time, but it will happen. Repetition is a power-ful force.

Don't go it alone. Seek out other people who are making healthy changes in their lives or who have already had success,

Dr. Martin suggests. You could join a weight-loss support group, seek out lunchtime walking buddies at work, or look to someone who's stopped smoking as a role model.

If your workout buddies are waiting for you at 12:30 every day, you may be more likely to go for your walk than if you had to do it alone. Having a role model can provide you with a reminder that people really *do* successfully change, and this person may be able to predict the bumps in the road that you're likely to encounter and help you get past them. (By the way, if you're trying to quit smoking, literally millions of Americans are former smokers, so they're not hard to find.)

Reward yourself. Our end payoff for all these changes is to be healthier in the future, with more money in our savings accounts that we didn't have to spend on medications, doctors, and hospitals. But you'll need earlier rewards than that to keep you inspired. Treat yourself to a small prize every time you hit a small goal: perhaps you can get a massage when you lose ten pounds, or a new MP3 player when you finish a five-kilometer race in under thirty minutes, or a three-day weekend trip when you get your blood pressure down to your target.

Recover from lapses. It's extremely common to veer from your new path. A cigarette here, a few trips through the fast-food drive-through there, or a missed week of exercise every once in a while. It's also common to feel like giving up after these little mishaps. "The big problem that I see is that once people take something on, if they have a small lapse, they say 'I failed.' That's a huge thing," Dr. Martin says.

Over a lifetime, these lapses are bound to happen, and you should see them as brief detours rather than an exit sign. One way to do this, Dr. Martin suggests, is to keep a record to track your progress over time. Whatever your new behavior is, jot down each day how well you've stuck to it. If you're exercising more, log your time or mileage. If you're cutting down on desserts, write down how many you've had. If you have a moment of weakness, you can look back over your records and say "Hmm . . . at least I stuck to the plan better this month than last month. I'm okay—let's continue."

Your New Prescription:

✓ Remember that emotional issues can affect your physical
  health, and vice versa. If you're bothered by nagging issues
  like headaches, back pain, fatigue, and difficulty sleeping,
  discuss with your healthcare provider whether your mood or
  emotions may be playing a role.

✓ While it's wise to put the appropriate amount of energy into
  taking care of your body, it's possible to be *too* focused on
  your health or health problems. If the time you spend worrying about your health or investigating health issues online is
  causing you distress, it may be time to think about whether
  you're inappropriately anxious about your health.

✓ Make choices each day that support your long-term health
  rather than jeopardize it. These choices must be *sustain-
  able*, meaning you can do them for a long period. A crash
  diet that helps you temporarily lose weight isn't the answer.
  Neither is diving into an extreme exercise program that
  you can't maintain. Make many small changes, with small
  goals, and develop many new habits that you enjoy and can
  sustain over the long haul. Surround yourself with support
  and lay the groundwork for lifestyle changes—like quitting
  smoking—rather than starting without a plan. If you have

an off day or let your healthy habits lapse for a while, pick them back up rather than quitting for good. But whatever you do, don't keep putting off changes you should make to improve your health.

8

Keep Your Money, Enjoy Your Better Health

While we were writing the book, one of us (Eric) was discussing the premise of our approach with a fellow alum from his university. The young woman mentioned that even though she and her husband both had health coverage through their employers, they still had run up five figures' worth of out-of-pocket medical expenses just for 2010.

"Needless to say, $23,000 will put a little dent in your finances," she noted with some understatement, "and it has taught me to really scrutinize every aspect of our healthcare costs." Since then, she has learned how to seek out bargains on medications, pick apart medical bills and call attention to suspicious charges, haggle over prices, and be a careful record keeper. In short, she's learned to put in the same work to find savings that people use when shopping for groceries, cars, houses, and other goods and services.

Most of our focus in this book has been on how patients can change their approach to using health care: being more critical when deciding which services you need, preventing disease when possible rather than hoping to cure it when it occurs, and taking the reins on decisions as appropriate rather than leaving them solely up to healthcare providers. We thought that this general approach could save you more money over the long haul—while leading to better health care and better health—rather than putting the focus on specific tips on saving money in specific situations.

However, making the right moves in certain situations can allow you to tuck back $10 here, $100 there, and much, much more in some circumstances. So let's take time to review some specific nuts-and-bolts methods for saving your healthcare dollars.

Consider Generics when Possible

According to the Food and Drug Administration (FDA), 70 percent of prescriptions filled in the United States are for generic drugs. These can be an easy way to save considerable money on your monthly health expenses. However, if you're hesitant to buy off-brand items in the supermarket or clothing store, it's understandable if you're somewhat suspicious of the thought of taking generic medications.

What exactly are generic drugs? When a drug maker gets a patent for a new drug, that protection only lasts for a set number of years. During this time, only the company can make the drug. When the patent expires, other companies can create their own generic version, with FDA approval. The newcomers don't have the steep costs for devising the drug from scratch or running expensive commercials repeatedly on television.

According to the FDA, generics contain the same active ingredient as their brand-name counterpart, and they have to work the same way. However, inactive ingredients may differ and generics have to look different from the brand-name drug.

You can often get generics for a small fraction of what you'd pay for the brand name. Health insurers these days often require people to pay a greater copayment for brand-name drugs than for generics or cover a greater percentage of the charge. If you're taking the drug to control a chronic condition, the savings can be considerable over the years. In addition, people often quit taking their medications—or they don't take them properly—and a common reason for this lack of adherence is the cost of the drugs. As a result, generics may help lead to improved health if you're better able to stick with them because they're affordable.

When your doctor prescribes a medication, especially if you'll be taking it for an extended period, ask if a generic is available. If it's not, and you're interested in saving money, ask if a *different* drug that has a generic form would work equally as well for you.

However, when using a generic, take a few precautions to ensure that it's working effectively:

Be selective with generics. For some drugs (the list is small), there's not a lot of room between the dosage that's needed to be effective and a dosage that can cause harm. In these cases, sticking with the brand name may be wise. Ask your doctor if your medication could be reasonably replaced with a generic or if it is better to remain with the brand name.

Keep tabs on your symptoms. The media has called attention in recent years to a number of cases in which individuals noted symptoms after they switched from a brand-name to a generic drug. If you notice that your symptoms get worse or new symptoms start occurring shortly after you begin taking a generic medication, talk to your doctor about it. Similarly, if you're taking drugs long term for issues such as high blood pressure or blood sugar and you keep track of your measurements, look back over these readings and see if they changed around the time you began taking the generic. These findings aren't always due to the switch, but they're worth bringing to your doctor's attention.

Get More Help with Medications

Americans spent an estimated $246 billion on prescription drugs in 2009, and spending on drugs is expected to grow by more than 5 percent in the near future, according to the Centers for Medicare & Medicaid Services. As a result, it's wise to explore a variety of ways to save money on prescriptions, in addition to using generics. Here are a few suggestions.

Be careful with samples. Your doctor may be able to provide free samples of medications that she has available in her office. If you only have a short-term problem, a supply of samples may be all you need to treat the condition. However, if you're going to be taking the medication for an extended period, starting out on a free sample may not be to your advantage. Doctors typically have free samples of newer, more expensive drugs, and once your sample runs out, you may be paying extra for this drug or need to switch to a cheaper one. Remember: there's no free lunch.

Seek help from drugmakers. Pharmaceutical companies often offer assistance programs for people who have difficulty affording medications. If you're truly in a financial position that leaves you needing a hand with a prescription, check out the website of the drug's maker to see if it has a program. Many of these allow you to apply online or over the phone.

You may also be able to find help through the Partnership for Prescription Assistance program, which helps low-income people find free or low-cost prescriptions through patient assistance programs. You can also find out more information about this program online at http://www.pparx.org/en/prescription_assistance_programs.

Stick to the plan . . . It's important to take your medications as they were intended. While taking a pill every other day will make a prescription last longer, your medication may no longer help you as it should—and it could even be harmful. This is not an efficient or cost-effective way to save money on your prescriptions.

. . . But review your meds from time to time. Sometimes a medication that used to be helpful becomes less so, or different doctors put you on different medications that are redundant or don't work well together, or a new medicine comes along that's a better choice. As a result, it's a good idea to occasionally review your medications with your doctor to make sure you're not taking any that could be halted. However, this is a choice to make *together*—not on your own.

Just talk about it. We've discussed how nonadherence is a common problem among Americans who take medications, particularly long term. This is an issue that doctors are aware of, and if we and our patients are going to take the time to treat a medical problem, we doctors really would like the patients to get the full benefit of the treatment.

So if you suspect that you're going to have trouble sticking to a drug because of its cost, let your doctor know up front. A good doctor would rather solve this problem right away than waste everyone's time with an approach that's doomed from the outset—and have your health worsen later because you couldn't afford a medication.

Consider Bringing in Help

Medical billing advocates appear to be growing in popularity. These businesses will step in and help you respond to your insurance company when it's not willing to cover a medical problem or a hospital or other medical provider if charges don't seem accurate.

Given the complexity of medical charges and the arcane rules by which the big players in the healthcare industry operate, having someone familiar with the nuts and bolts of the system can help you save considerable money if you're injured in an accident or develop an expensive illness. With staff members coming from careers in insurance companies or hospitals, Kevin Flynn, president of Healthcare Advocates in Philadelphia, likens his business to the IRS. But instead of auditing taxpayers and finding errors in their calculations, they analyze hospital bills and health insurers' documents for problems. Not only can an experienced professional find errors in the dense columns of numbers on a medical bill, simply having an advocate on your side can lead to a quicker and more satisfying response than if you tried to deal with the company on your own, he points out.

Billing advocates may charge you a flat fee, an hourly rate, or a portion of the money they save you. Candy Butcher, CEO of Medical Billing Associates of America, says their advocates' business is split about evenly between insured and uninsured customers. "There's definitely a lack of education among consumers," she says. "Many people who call don't realize they have rights. You *can* question medical bills. You *can* request an uninsured discount. If something is denied by your insurance and you feel it's something that should have been paid, you do have the option of appeal."

It's beyond the scope of this book to teach you every method of finding errors or prodding your insurer to cover more of your bills. But here are a few general suggestions to keep in mind that you may do on your own:

Appeal. If your insurance company tells you it's not covering a procedure or it's not covering it to the level that you think it should, appeal it, Butcher says. Simply providing a document from your provider that states that a treatment was medically necessary may be enough to reverse the insurer's decision. Just keep in mind that their initial denial is not the final answer, she says. You have the potential to change it.

Call ahead. If you're planning to have a surgery or other expensive procedure, do your homework to ensure that *all* your providers are within your health insurers' network. Don't just check to make sure that the hospital is within the network—also check the surgeon, anesthesia provider, radiologist, pathologist, physical therapists, and other professionals who'll be handling your care, Butcher recommends. "We see that all the time: A lot of consumers say, 'I went to an in-network hospital, but I'm getting bills saying I owe them $10,000.' Come to find out, [some of the services] were out of network and the majority of that bill is due to the difference between the total bill and the amount allowed by the insurance company."

If it's an emergency, this will be harder to do. Although a lot of other stuff is going on, if a friend or family members are with you, they should check with admissions and try to make sure that all providers are covered within your health insurer's network, she recommends.

Ask for help. If you're uninsured and need surgery, ask if the hospital will offer an uninsured discount, Butcher says. Hospitals may be willing to deduct a chunk right off the top. If your income is low enough, you may qualify for charitable assistance. Be sure to fill out the forms carefully and follow up on them before you go in for the procedure to ensure that you qualify for the assistance and will indeed receive it.

Request an itemized statement. "The number one tip for consumers is to ask for an itemized statement from the hospital," Butcher says. If you've had a surgery or other expensive procedure, a summary bill may bundle a number of charges together for one fee, say, $20,000 for miscellaneous supplies. An itemized bill will break them down and give you a better sense of where to look for discrepancies.

For example, a hospital may charge by the minute for your time in the operating room. "That fee includes anything standard for that operating room for every procedure, for every patient," Butcher says. "You'll notice on that detailed itemized statement the gloves, drapes, sutures, and scissors—just numerous supplies. On an itemized statement, sometimes you'll see those billed for separately when they should have been included in that room rate. When we see those, we consider those nonbillable." In some cases, these charges may have already been factored in the price per sixty seconds for the use of that room, she adds.

In addition, check your charges for details like how long the anesthesia provider billed for his or her services, Flynn recommends. Does it correspond with the length of your surgery? And check the codes on your bill. These include CPT codes (which stands for Current Procedural Terminology) and ICD codes (which stands for International Classification of Diseases). CPT codes describe procedures that a provider does, ranging from checking lab values of your blood to major operations. An ICD code describes your precise diagnosis. You can look up CPT and ICD codes online to see if they seem reasonable. For example, providers may get paid more to treat one condition as opposed to another that's similar. A check of your ICD code may find that you were treated for a problem that you don't really have, Flynn says.

"There's an art form" to this kind of homework, he goes on to say, which requires careful attention and some practice, so if you're ever thinking about making use of a billing advocate, this may be one of the jobs that would most benefit from extra expertise.

But you too can learn the expertise and use it for your protection. The young woman we mentioned at the beginning of the chapter notes: "I've learned to look up medical billing/diagnostic codes online—and sometimes I don't agree. When I don't and it makes the difference between coverage and no insurance coverage, I call the doctor's office or hospital and question the diagnostic code. I've caught blatant coding errors and I've saved about $3,000 doing this."

Do some end-of-the-year housekeeping. At the end of the year—in December or so—ask your insurance company for a history printout of the past year, Butcher recommends. This will show you every claim that the insurer received on you or your family throughout the year. She's found that billing advocates often see that consumers wound up exceeding their out of pocket limits for the year.

"From your history printout, say if your out-of-pocket was $2,500 and you noticed that you paid $3,500 out-of-pocket, call the company. They'll go back and research it and if it's accurate, normally they'll send a check to the patient," she notes.

Get the Right Health Coverage for Your Needs

Make a priority of having health insurance. Yes, it can be expensive, but even going without coverage for a month can be financially devastating if an accident occurs or major health condition develops during that period.

Be sure that your health insurance covers your current needs, and if possible your needs for the immediate future. Are you a young, healthy, single person who rarely gets sick and doesn't take any medications? Perhaps a plan with a high deductible is right for you. If you have chronic conditions and take several medications, you may be better served by a plan with a lower deductible and reasonable copays and out-of-pocket costs. If you're insured through your job, talk to your human resources representative or other staffer who handles benefits to make sure you're making the choice that best fits your needs.

Shop Around

If you're uninsured, it's in your best interest to shop around when you need either routine or major health services. The market seems to be providing more opportunities for patients who are paying out of pocket to make deals with providers.

In recent years, consumers have shown a greater willingness to go out of their way to find a bargain on medical services. Just witness the rise of medical tourism. In 2007, an estimated 750,000 Americans traveled abroad for medical treatment, a number that was expected to rise to 6 million by 2010.

Depending on where they live and the country offering the surgery, patients may save up to 90 percent on procedures. Common medical-tourism destinations include Mexico, Costa Rica, Brazil, India, and Singapore.

I'm *not* recommending that people travel overseas for their medical care, however, as I'm far more familiar and comfortable with the level of care available here in the United States. However, the mere existence of overseas medical tourism may actually help consumers find lower costs in the United States in a roundabout way.

Administrators in some American hospitals have taken note of patients' willingness to travel far from home for their surgeries—and to pay cash. One company that arranges overseas medical-tourism trips for patients has recently begun setting up deals with domestic healthcare providers. Such hospitals are now offering discounted surgeries, especially during weekends and other low-volume times. Even after steeply cutting costs, a hospital can still make a profit on a surgery when the operating table and surgical equipment would otherwise have been idle.

You may also save by finding a primary doctor who caters primarily to cash-paying patients. According to an article in the *U.S. News & World Report*, in mid-2009, hundreds of family medicine practices across the country had gone cash-only. These practices typically draw in patients without insurance or those with high-deductible plans that are better used for major illnesses or injuries. In this type of setup, the cost of your visits may be more clear and up front—for example, ten-, twenty-, or thirty-minute visits may each cost a certain amount. These types of practices may be worth investigating.

However, if you're uninsured, you enjoy your current physician, and you don't wish to start up a relationship with another, ask if you can have a discount for paying cash. The doctor's office may work with you to set up a plan.

In coming years, you may also find more doctors and hospitals using new techniques to reach out to patients with discount services, which brings us to our final *New Prescription* for getting the health care you need at a price you can afford.

A New System Brings New Chances for Savings

For all the good our healthcare system accomplishes—for all the lives saved from the brink of death, for the good quality of life it can provide in the face of illness—it really hasn't offered a level playing field for the consumers it serves.

When they get sick, people often seem to be at the mercy of the big players in health care. Health insurers have wielded great power in setting the rules. Hospitals can generate the largest bill that people have ever seen in their lives after just a relatively short stay. You may wait thirty minutes or more to see a doctor for a ten-minute visit. You may have had to make a life-changing decision too quickly and with insufficient information.

Traditionally, consumers haven't held much clout in their interactions with healthcare providers. It's been difficult to shop around to find the best price for medical procedures beforehand. It's been a challenge to find out which procedure is best, or if *any* procedure is even necessary. The coauthors of this book can't think of many other situations—if any—in which consumers have to spend big money on a vital product while having so little control over its cost or knowledge about what they're buying.

But we think that's changing.

In the coming days, months, and years, we suspect that all sorts of tools are going to enter the marketplace to help consumers become better-informed purchasers of health services at a good value.

While we were putting this book together, we learned about a website that works a bit like the familiar online service that lets you offer your own price for a hotel room, which the hotel may accept. It focuses on elective procedures ranging from tummy tucks and nose reshaping to colonoscopies, and it's geared toward patients who are uninsured or underinsured. We found another company that acts as a go-between for patients who need surgeries (and who are willing to travel in the United States for them) and hospitals that are willing to provide those surgeries at a discount.

We found a website—Healthcare Blue Book at www.health carebluebook.com—that offers a crucial piece of information that has historically been difficult to find: how much you can expect to pay for surgeries, lab tests, and other diagnostic and treatment procedures in your area. We're also excited about the national push for comparative effectiveness research, which will weigh treatments for specific medical problems against one another to see which ones offer the best chance for good results. Hopefully this information will get passed along to the public in a form that's easy to access, understand, and use when making decisions.

Times are changing, and so is the way you purchase health-care products and services. Keep your eyes open for healthcare-related discount programs and online shopping services as they become more available. Take a critical approach to weighing your options when your doctor suggests a medical treatment. Talk to your friends about how *they've* saved money on health care. Don't accept a given price for health care as the final number. Make your own offers.

In short, put as much time and attention into your healthcare purchases as you do clipping coupons before a trip to the super-market or doing your homework before buying a car or a home-entertainment system. As the healthcare system slowly evolves, opportunities to gain more power will drift into your grasp. Stay ready to make use of them.

The *old* prescription of giving doctors, hospitals, and the rest of the healthcare system all the responsibility for your health care is out-of-date. That approach was too costly and too often delivered unsatisfactory results. The healthcare system is facing a crisis. It's badly in need of reform. And it's facing big changes in our lifetimes.

Good. It's overdue for a big change. And you as a health consumer (and seeker of health) probably are ready for a change, too.

The *new* prescription you've just received gives you new opportunities and new responsibilities. It's time to pay less for health care *and* expect better results. It's time to speak up more, ask more questions, and know more about the options that are available to you.

You have the tools and the knowledge. Now it's time to use them. Good luck as you seek better health for yourself . . . and your bank account.

Bibliography

Abbo, E., et al. "The Increasing Number of Clinical Items Addressed During the Time of Adult Primary Care Visits." *Journal of General Internal Medicine* 23 (2008): 2058–2065.

Ablin, R. "The Great Prostate Mistake." *New York Times,* March 9, 2010, http://www.nytimes.com/2010/03/10/opinion/10Ablin.html.

Adami, H. "The Prostate Cancer Pseudo-Epidemic." *Acta Oncologica* 49 (2010): 298–304.

Agency for Healthcare Research and Quality. "20 Tips to Help Prevent Medical Errors." http://www.ahrq.gov/consumer/20tips.htm.

———. "Big Money: Cost of 10 Most Expensive Health Conditions Near $500 Billion." http://www.ahrq.gov/news/nn/nn012308.htm.

———. "The High Concentration of U.S. Health Care Expenditures." http://www.ahrq.gov/research/ria19/expendria.htm#HowAre.

———. "Medical Expenditure Panel Survey." http://www.meps.ahrq.gov/mepsweb/data_stats/tables_compendia_hh_interactive.jsp?_SERVICE=MEPSSocket0&_PROGRAM=MEPSPGM.TC.SAS&File=HCFY2007&Table=HCFY2007_PLEXP_E&VAR1=AGE&VAR2=SEX&VAR3=RACETH5C&VAR4=INSURCOV&VAR5=POVCAT07&VAR6=MSA&VAR7=REGION&VAR8=HEALTH&.

———. "Primary Care Doctors Account for Nearly Half of Physician Visits but Less than One-Third of Expenses." http://www.ahrq.gov/news/nn/nn042507.htm.

Alzheimer's Association. "2010 Alzheimer's Disease Facts and Figures." http://www.alz.org/documents_custom/report_alzfactsfigures2010.pdf.

American Academy of Family Physicians. "Charts and Graphs." http://www.aafp.org/online/en/home/media/charts-and-graphs.html.

———. "Questions and Answers on Acute Otitis Media." http://www.aafp.org/online/etc/medialib/aafp_org/documents/clinical/clin_recs/acute_otitis_media.Par.0001.File.dat/aom_qanda.pdf.

American Academy of Pediatrics. "Clinical Practice Guideline: Diagnosis and Management of Acute Otitis Media." *Pediatrics* 113 (2004): 1451–1465.

American Academy of Orthopaedic Surgeons. "Home Safety Checklist." http://orthoinfo. aaos.org/topic.cfm?topic=A00123.

American Cancer Society. "ACS Guidelines on Nutrition and Physical Activity for Cancer Prevention."http://www.cancer.org/Healthy/EatHealthyGetActive/ACSGuidelineson NutritionPhysicalActivityforCancerPrevention/acs-guidelines-on-nutrition-and-physical-activity-for-cancer-prevention-intro.

———. "American Cancer Society Guidelines for the Early Detection of Cancer." http:// www.cancer.org/Healthy/FindCancerEarly/CancerScreeningGuidelines/american-cancer-society-guidelines-for-the-early-detection-of-cancer.

———. "Can Prostate Cancer Be Found Early?" http://www.cancer.org/Cancer/Prostate Cancer/DetailedGuide/prostate-cancer-detection.

———. "Cancer Facts and Figures 2010." http://www.cancer.org/acs/groups/content/@ nho/documents/document/acspc-024113.pdf.

———."CigaretteSmoking."http://www.cancer.org/Cancer/CancerCauses/TobaccoCancer/ CigaretteSmoking/cigarette-smoking-who-and-how-affects-health.

———. "Common Questions About Diet and Cancer." http://ww2.cancer.org/docroot/ PED/content/PED_3_2X_Common_Questions_About_Diet_and_Cancer.asp.

———. "Guide to Quitting Smoking." http://www.cancer.org/Healthy/StayAwayfrom Tobacco/GuidetoQuittingSmoking/guide-to-quitting-smoking-how-to-quit.

———. "Guide to Quitting Smoking." http://www.cancer.org/acs/groups/cid/documents/ webcontent/002971-pdf.pdf.

———. "Lycopene." http://www.cancer.org/Treatment/TreatmentsandSideEffects/Com plementaryandAlternativeMedicine/DietandNutrition/lycopene.

———."SecondhandSmoke."http://www.cancer.org/Cancer/CancerCauses/TobaccoCancer/ secondhand-smoke.

———. "Skin Cancer Prevention and Early Detection." http://www.cancer.org/docroot/ ped/content/ped_7_1_skin_cancer_detection_what_you_can_do.asp.

American Cancer Society and LIVESTRONG. "The Global Economic Cost of Cancer." http://www.cancer.org/acs/groups/content/@internationalaffairs/documents/ document/acspc-026203.pdf.

American College of Physicians. "Reform of the Dysfunctional Healthcare Payment and Delivery System." http://www.acponline.org/advocacy/where_we_stand/policy/ dysfunctional_payment.pdf.

American Congress of Obstetricians and Gynecologists. "ACOG Practice Bulletin— Number 108: Polycystic Ovary Syndrome." *Obstetrics & Gynecology* 114 (2009): 936–949.

———. "First Cervical Cancer Screening Delayed Until Age 21; Less Frequent Pap Tests Recommended." http://www.acog.org/from_home/publications/press_releases/ nr11-20-09.cfm.

———. "Polycystic Ovary Syndrome." http://www.acog.org/publications/patienteducation/bp121.cfm.

———. "Screening Tests for Birth Defects." http://www.acog.org/publications/patient education/bp165.cfm.

American Dental Association. "Cleaning Your Teeth & Gums." http://www.ada.org/2624.aspx.

American Diabetes Association. "Diabetes Statistics." http://www.diabetes.org/diabetes-basics/diabetes-statistics/.

———. "Economic Costs of Diabetes in the U.S. in 2007." *Diabetes Care* 31 (2008): 596–615.

———. "Nutrition Recommendations and Interventions for Diabetes: A Position Statement of the American Diabetes Association." *Diabetes Care* 31 (2008): S61–78.

———. "Pre-Diabetes FAQs." http://www.diabetes.org/diabetes-basics/prevention/pre-diabetes/pre-diabetes-faqs.html.

American Health Information Management Association. "Helping Consumers Select PHRs: Questions and Considerations for Navigating an Emerging Market." http://library.ahima.org/xpedio/groups/public/documents/ahima/bok1_032260.hcsp?dDocName=bok1_032260.

American Heart Association. "Cardiovascular Disease Cost." http://www.americanheart.org/presenter.jhtml?identifier=4475.

———. "Heart Disease and Stroke Statistics—2010 Update." *Circulation* 121 (2010): e46–e215.

———. "Metabolic Syndrome." http://www.americanheart.org/presenter.jhtml?identifier=4756.

———. "Primary Prevention in the Adult." http://www.americanheart.org/presenter.jhtml?identifier=4704.

———. "Understand Your Risk of Heart Attack." http://www.americanheart.org/presenter.jhtml?identifier=4726.

———. "Whole Grains and Fiber." http://www.americanheart.org/presenter.jhtml?identifier=4574.

American Pregnancy Association. "First Trimester Screen." http://www.americanpregnancy.org/prenataltesting/firstscreen.html.

American Society for Reproductive Medicine. "Frequently Asked Questions About Infertility." http://www.asrm.org/awards/index.aspx?id=3012.

Anderson, G. "Chronic Care: Making the Case for Ongoing Care." Robert Wood Johnson Foundation. http://www.rwjf.org/files/research/50968chronic.care.chartbook.pdf.

Anderson, J. "Save Money on Prescriptions." Kiplinger, May 2008. http://www.kiplinger.com/magazine/archives/2008/05/reduce-prescription-drug-costs.html.

Anderson, J. L., et al. "Patient Information Recall in a Rheumatology Clinic." *Rheumatology and Rehabilitation* 18 (1979): 18–22.

Andriole, G., et al. "Mortality Results from a Randomized Prostate Cancer Screening Trial." *New England Journal of Medicine* 360 (2009): 1310–1319.

Anstey, K., et al. "Smoking as a Risk Factor for Dementia and Cognitive Decline: A Meta-Analysis of Prospective Studies." *American Journal of Epidemiology* 166 (2007): 367–378.

Arbyn, M., et al. "Perinatal Mortality and Other Severe Adverse Pregnancy Outcomes Associated with Treatment of Cervical Intraepithelial Neoplasia: Meta-Analysis." *BMJ* 337 (2008): a1284.

Associated Press. "Bush Undergoes Annual Physical Exam." *USA Today*, August 1, 2006, http://www.usatoday.com/news/washington/2006-08-01-bush-physical_x.htm.

———. "Obama Hasn't Kicked Smoking, But in 'Excellent Health.'" *New York Post*, February 28, 2010, http://www.nypost.com/p/news/politics/obama_checkup_excellent_ health_still_p4cnqNMCY3VineErslej4I.

Atkin, W., et al. "Once-Only Flexible Sigmoidoscopy Screening in Prevention of Colorectal Cancer: A Multicentre Randomised Controlled Trial." *Lancet* 375 (2010): 1624–1633.

Azziz, R., et al. "Health Care-Related Economic Burden of the Polycystic Ovary Syndrome During the Reproductive Life Span." *Journal of Clinical Endocrinology & Metabolism* 90 (2005): 4650–4658.

Badley, E., et al. "Arthritis and Arthritis-Attributable Activity Limitations in the United States and Canada: A Cross-Border Comparison." *Arthritis & Rheumatism* 62 (2010): 308–315.

Bailey, S., et al. "A Simulation Model Investigating the Impact of Tumor Volume Doubling Time and Mammographic Tumor Detectability on Screening Outcomes in Women Aged 40–49 Years." *Journal of the National Cancer Institute* 102 (2010): 1263–1271.

Baron, R. "What's Keeping Us So Busy in Primary Care?" *New England Journal of Medicine* 362 (2010): 1632–1636.

Barsky, A., et al. "Somatization Increases Medical Utilization and Costs Independent of Psychiatric and Medical Comorbidity." *Archives of General Psychiatry* 62 (2005): 903–910.

Bartlett, S. "Role of Body Weight in Osteoarthritis." Johns Hopkins Arthritis Center. http://www.hopkins-arthritis.org/patient-corner/disease-management/osteoand weight.html.

Bernstein, A., et al. "Major Dietary Protein Sources and Risk of Coronary Heart Disease in Women." *Circulation* 122 (2010): 876–883.

Bezakova, N., et al. "Recurrence Up to 3.5 Years After Antibiotic Treatment of Acute Otitis Media in Very Young Dutch Children: Survey of Trial Participants." *BMJ* 338 (2009): b2525.

Bicyclinginfo.org. "Bike Safely." http://www.bicyclinginfo.org/bikemore/safely.cfm.

Borghouts, L., et al. "Exercise and Insulin Sensitivity: A Review." *International Journal of Sports Medicine* 21 (2000): 1–12.

Brawley, O. "Prostate Cancer Screening: Is This a Teachable Moment?" *Journal of the National Cancer Institute* 101 (2009): 1295–1297.

Brody, H. "Medicine's Ethical Responsibility for Health Care Reform—The Top Five List." *New England Journal of Medicine* 362 (2010): 283–285.

Brown, D., et al. "Projected Costs of Ischemic Stroke in the United States." *Neurology* 67 (2006): 1390–1395.

Brown, S. "Medical Tourism: Nations Vie for Health Dollars," *Hospitals & Health Networks.* http://www.hhnmag.com/hhnmag_app/jsp/articledisplay.jsp?dcrpath=HHNMAG/Article/data/12DEC2008/0812HHN_Scope_DataPage&domain=HHNMAG.

Cade, J., et al. "Dietary Fibre and Risk of Breast Cancer in the UK Women's Cohort Study." *International Journal of Epidemiology* 36 (2007): 431–438.

Calle, E., et al. "Overweight, Obesity, and Mortality from Cancer in a Prospectively Studied Cohort of U.S. Adults." *New England Journal of Medicine* 348 (2003): 1625–1638.

Carney, P., et al. "Individual and Combined Effects of Age, Breast Density and Hormone Replacement Therapy Use on the Accuracy of Mammography." *Annals of Internal Medicine* 138 (2003): 168–175.

Carter, P., et al. "Fruit and Vegetable Intake and Incidence of Type 2 Diabetes Mellitus: Systematic Review and Meta-Analysis." *BMJ* 341 (2010): c4229. Online First: http://www.bmj.com/content/341/bmj.c4229.full.pdf+html.

Catalona, W. J., et al. "Measurement of Prostate-Specific Antigen in Serum as a Screening Test for Prostate Cancer." *New England Journal of Medicine* 324 (1991): 1156–1161.

Centers for Disease Control and Prevention. "Arthritis-Related Statistics." http://www.cdc.gov/arthritis/data_statistics/arthritis_related_stats.htm.

———. "Fertility, Family Planning, and Reproductive Health of U.S. Women: Data from the 2002 National Survey of Family Growth." http://www.cdc.gov/nchs/data/series/sr_23/sr23_025.pdf.

———. "Genital HPV Infection." http://www.cdc.gov/std/hpv/stdfact-hpv.htm#howget.

———. "Health Insurance Coverage: Early Release of Estimates from the National Health Interview Survey, January–June 2009." http://www.cdc.gov/nchs/data/nhis/earlyrelease/insur200912.htm.

———. "Key Facts About Influenza (Flu) & Flu Vaccine." http://www.cdc.gov/flu/keyfacts.htm#whoshould1.

———. "Key Facts About Seasonal Flu Vaccine." http://www.cdc.gov/flu/protect/keyfacts.htm.

———. "Leading Causes of Death." http://www.cdc.gov/nchs/fastats/lcod.htm.

———. "NCHS Data on Prescription Drugs." http://www.cdc.gov/nchs/data/factsheets/factsheet_prescription_drugs.htm.

———. "Obesity and Overweight." http://www.cdc.gov/nchs/fastats/overwt.htm.

———. "Pelvic Inflammatory Disease—CDC Fact Sheet." http://www.cdc.gov/std/pid/stdfact-pid.htm.

————. "Pneumococcal Disease—In Short." http://www.cdc.gov/vaccines/vpd-vac/pneumo/in-short-both.htm.

————. "Seasonal Influenza." http://www.cdc.gov/flu/about/qa/disease.htm.

————. "Stopping Germs at Home, Work and School." http://www.cdc.gov/germstopper/home_work_school.htm.

Centers for Medicare and Medicaid Services. "National Health Expenditure Projections, 2009–2019." http://www.cms.gov/NationalHealthExpendData/downloads/proj2009.pdf.

Chen, L., et al. "Primary Care Visit Duration and Quality: Does Good Care Take Longer?" *Archives of Internal Medicine* 169 (2009): 1866–1872.

Chernew, M., et al. "Would Having More Primary Care Doctors Cut Health Spending Growth?" *Health Affairs* 28 (2009): 1327–1335.

Christensen, A., et al. "Patient and Physician Beliefs About Control over Health: Association of Symmetrical Beliefs with Medication Regimen Adherence." *Journal of General Internal Medicine* 25 (2010): 397–402.

Claxton, G., et al. "Health Benefits in 2008: Premiums Moderately Higher, While Enrollment in Consumer-Directed Plans Rises in Small Firms." *Health Affairs* 27 (2008): 492–502.

Cohen, D. L., et al. "Iyengar Yoga versus Enhanced Usual Care on Blood Pressure in Patients with Prehypertension to Stage I Hypertension: A Randomized Controlled Trial." *Evidence-Based Complementary and Alternative Medicine,* eCAM Advance Access published September 4, 2009. http://ecam.oxfordjournals.org/cgi/reprint/nep130v1.

Conrad, Peter. *The Medicalization of Society.* Baltimore: Johns Hopkins University Press, 2007.

Conrad, P., et al. "Estimating the Costs of Medicalization." *Social Science & Medicine* 70 (2010): 1943–1947.

Cooner, W., et al. "Prostate Cancer Detection in a Clinical Urological Practice by Ultrasonography, Digital Rectal Examination and Prostate Specific Antigen." *Journal of Urology* 143 (1990): 1146–1152.

Costanzo, S., et al. "Alcohol Consumption and Mortality in Patients with Cardiovascular Disease: A Meta-Analysis." *Journal of the American College of Cardiology* 55 (2010): 1339–1347.

Cross, A., et al. "A Prospective Study of Red and Processed Meat Intake in Relation to Cancer Risk." *PLoS Medicine* 4 (2007).

Dahm, C. C., et al. "Dietary Fiber and Colorectal Cancer Risk: A Nested Case-Control Study Using Food Diaries." *Journal of the National Cancer Institute* 102 (2010): 614–626.

Danaei, G., et al. "The Preventable Causes of Death in the United States: Comparative Risk Assessment of Dietary, Lifestyle, and Metabolic Risk Factors." *PLoS Medicine* 6 (2009).

Dartmouth Institute for Health Policy & Clinical Practice. "Tracking the Care of Patients with Severe Chronic Illness: The Dartmouth Atlas of Health Care 2008." http://www.dartmouthatlas.org/downloads/atlases/2008_Chronic_Care_Atlas.pdf.

Davidson, K. "Don't Worry, Be Happy: Positive Affect and Reduced 10-Year Incident of Coronary Heart Disease; The Canadian Nova Scotia Health Survey." *European Heart Journal* 31 (2010): 1065–1070.

Deloitte Center for Health Solutions. "Medical Tourism: Consumers in Search of Value." http://www.deloitte.com/assets/Dcom-UnitedStates/Local%20Assets/Documents/us_chs_MedicalTourismStudy(3).pdf.

Denollet, J. "Anger, Suppressed Anger, and Risk of Adverse Events in Patients with Coronary Artery Disease." *American Journal of Cardiology* 105 (2010): 1555–1560.

Diabetes Prevention Program Research Group. "Reduction in the Incidence of Type 2 Diabetes with Lifestyle Intervention or Metformin." *New England Journal of Medicine* 346 (2002): 393–403.

———. "10-year Follow-up of Diabetes Incidence and Weight Loss in the Diabetes Prevention Program Outcomes Study." *Lancet* 374 (2009): 1677–1686.

Dodge, J., et al. "Lumen Diameter of Normal Human Coronary Arteries: Influence of Age, Sex, Anatomic Variation, and Left Ventricular Hypertrophy or Dilation." *Circulation* 86 (1992): 232–246.

Donaldson, M., et al. *Primary Care: America's Health in a New Era.* Washington, DC: National Academies Press, 1996.

Elkin, E., et al. "Cancer's Next Frontier Addressing High and Increasing Costs." *Journal of the American Medical Association* 303 (2010): 1086–1087.

Elliott, V. "'Speed Dating' Matches Physicians, Patients." American Medical News. http://www.ama-assn.org/amednews/2010/02/08/bil20208.htm.

Emanuel, E., et al. "The Perfect Storm of Overutilization." *Journal of the American Medical Association* 299 (2008): 2789–2791.

Emerging Risk Factors Collaboration. "Diabetes Mellitus, Fasting Blood Glucose Concentration, and Risk of Vascular Disease: A Collaborative Meta-Analysis of 102 Prospective Studies." *Lancet* 375:2215–2222.

Employee Benefit Research Institute. "Savings Needed to Fund Health Insurance and Health Care Expenses in Retirement: Findings from a Simulation Model." http://www.ebri.org/pdf/EBRI_IB_05-2008.pdf.

Escobar, J., et al. "Somatization in the Community: Relationship to Disability and Use of Services." *American Journal of Public Health* 77 (1987): 837–840.

Feart, C., et al. "Mediterranean Diet and Cognitive Function in Older Adults." *Current Opinion in Clinical Nutrition and Metabolic Care* 13 (2010): 14–18.

Federal Trade Commission. "Prescription Assistance Programs." http://www.ftc.gov/bcp/edu/microsites/whocares/prescriptionassist.shtm.

Fendrick, A., et al. "The Economic Burden of Non-Influenza-Related Viral Respiratory Tract Infection in the United States." *Archives of Internal Medicine* 163 (2003): 487–494.

Finkelstein, E., et al. "The Lifetime Medical Cost Burden of Overweight and Obesity: Implications for Obesity Prevention." *Obesity* 16 (2008): 1843–1848.

Finkelstein, E., et al. "Annual Medical Spending Attributable to Obesity: Payer- and Service-Specific Estimates." *Health Affairs* 28 (2009): 822–831.

Finkelstein, E., et al. "The Personal Financial Burden of Cancer for the Working-Aged Population." *American Journal of Managed Care* 15 (2009): 801–806.

Fisher, E., et al. "Slowing the Growth of Health Care Costs—Lessons from Regional Variation." *New England Journal of Medicine* 360 (2009): 849–852.

Fishman J., et al. "Cancer and the Media: How Does the News Report on Treatment and Outcomes?" *Archives of Internal Medicine* 170 (2010): 515–518.

Galeone, C., et al. "Onion and Garlic Use and Human Cancer." *American Journal of Clinical Nutrition* 84 (2006): 1027–1032.

Galewitz, P. "Health Bills in Congress Won't Fix Doctor Shortage." Kaiser Health News. http://www.kaiserhealthnews.org/Stories/2009/October/12/primary-care-doctor-shortage.aspx.

Gawande, A. "The Cost Conundrum: What a Texas Town Can Teach Us About Health Care." *New Yorker*, June 1, 2009, http://www.newyorker.com/reporting/2009/06/01/090601fa_fact_gawande.

Giuliano, J. "Can You Legally Refuse to Hire Someone Who Smokes?" HR Morning, February 16, 2010, http://www.hrmorning.com/can-you-legally-refuse-to-hire-someone-who-smokes/.

Harris Interactive. "Nearly Half of Americans Worried About Rising Health-Care Costs." http://www.harrisinteractive.com/NewsRoom/PressReleases/tabid/446/mid/1506/articleId/49/ctl/ReadCustom%20Default/Default.aspx.

HealthCare.gov. "Timeline: What's Changing and When." http://www.healthcare.gov/law/timeline/.

HealthyPeople2010. "HealthCommunication." http://www.healthypeople.gov/document/html/volume1/11healthcom.htm.

Higdon, J., et al. "Cruciferous Vegetables and Human Cancer Risk: Epidemiologic Evidence and Mechanistic Basis." *Pharmacological Research* 55 (2007): 224–236.

Himmelstein, D., et al. "Medical Bankruptcy in the United States, 2007: Results of a National Study." *American Journal of Medicine* 122 (2009): 741–746.

Hugosson, J. "Mortality Results from the Göteborg Randomised Population-Based Prostate-Cancer Screening Trial." *Lancet Oncology* 11 (2010): 725–732.

Institute of Medicine. "To Err Is Human: Building a Safer Health System." http://www.iom.edu/~/media/Files/Report%20Files/1999/To-Err-is-Human/To%20Err%20is%20Human%201999%20%20report%20brief.ashx.

Janiszewski, P., et al. "Does Waist Circumference Predict Diabetes and Cardiovascular Disease Beyond Commonly Evaluated Cardiometabolic Risk Factors?" *Diabetes Care* 30 (2007): 3105–3109.

Kahn, S., et al. "Obesity, Body Fat Distribution, Insulin Sensitivity and Islet Beta-Cell Function as Explanations for Metabolic Diversity." *Journal of Nutrition* 131 (2001): 354S–360S.

Kaiser Commission on Medicaid and the Uninsured. *The Distribution of Assets in the Elderly Population Living in the Community.* Washington, D.C.: Henry A. Kaiser Family Foundation, 2005.

Kaiser Family Foundation. "Prescription Drug Trends." http://www.kff.org/rxdrugs/upload/3057-08.pdf.

Kaiser State Health Facts. "Total Nurse Practitioners, 2009." http://www.statehealth facts.org/comparemaptable.jsp?ind=773&cat=8.

Kane, C. "Medical Liability Claim Frequency: A 2007–2008 Snapshot of Physicians." American Medical Association. http://www.ama-assn.org/ama1/pub/upload/mm/363/prp-201001-claim-freq.pdf.

Katz, M. "Failing the Acid Test: Benefits of Proton Pump Inhibitors May Not Justify the Risks for Many Users." *Archives of Internal Medicine* 170 (2010): 747–748.

Kelley Blue Book. "2010 Ford Fusion 4-door SEL Sedan." http://www.kbb.com/new-cars/ford/fusion/2010/pricing-report?id=248364.

Kelley, R. "Where Can $700 Billion in Waste Be Cut Annually from the US Healthcare System?" Thomson Reuters, October 2009.

Kessels, R. P. C. "Patients' Memory for Medical Information. *Journal of the Royal Society of Medicine* 96 (2003): 219–222.

Kim, M., et al. "How Interested Are Americans in New Medical Technologies? A Multi-country Comparison." *Health Affairs* 20 (2001): 194–201.

Kocurek, B. "Promoting Medication Adherence in Older Adults . . . and the Rest of Us." *Diabetes Spectrum* 22 (2009): 80–84.

Kolata, G. "Cancer Society, In Shift, Has Concerns on Screenings." *New York Times*, October 20, 2009, http://www.nytimes.com/2009/10/21/health/21cancer.html.

Koopman, R., et al. "Changes in Age at Diagnosis of Type 2 Diabetes Mellitus in the United States, 1988 to 2000." *Annals of Family Medicine* 3 (2005): 60–63.

Kotlarz, H., et al. "Insurer and Out-of-Pocket Costs of Osteoarthritis in the US." *Arthritis & Rheumatism* 60 (2009): 3546–3553.

Kravet, S., et al. "Health Care Utilization and the Proportion of Primary Care Physicians." *American Journal of Medicine* 121 (2008): 142–148.

Lewis, C., et al. "Patient Preferences for Care by General Internists and Specialists in the Ambulatory Setting." *Journal of General Internal Medicine* 15 (2000): 75–83.

Liao, L., et al. "Economic Burden of Heart Failure in the Elderly." *PharmacoEconomics* 26 (2008): 447–462.

Lindström, J., et al. "Sustained Reduction in the Incidence of Type 2 Diabetes by Lifestyle Intervention: Follow-up of the Finnish Diabetes Prevention Study." *Lancet* 368 (2006): 1673–1679.

Llewellyn, D., et al. "Exposure to Secondhand Smoke and Cognitive Impairment in Non-Smokers: National Cross Sectional Study with Cotinine Measurement." *BMJ* 338 (2009): b462.

Losina, E., et al. "Cost-effectiveness of Total Knee Arthroplasty in the United States." *Archives of Internal Medicine* 169 (2009): 1113–1121.

Lusardi, A., et al. "The Economic Crisis and Medical Care Usage." http://www.hbs.edu/research/pdf/10-079.pdf.

Malizia, B., et al. "Cumulative Live-Birth Rates after In Vitro Fertilization." *New England Journal of Medicine* 360 (2009): 236–243.

Mallya, G., et al. "Are Primary Care Physicians Ready to Practice in a Consumer-Driven Environment?" *American Journal of Managed Care* 14 (2008): 661–668.

Massachusetts Medical Society. "Investigation of Defensive Medicine in Massachusetts." http://www.massmed.org/AM/Template.cfm?Section=Research_Reports_and_Studies2&TEMPLATE=/CM/ContentDisplay cfm&CONTENTID=27797.

Mattioli, D. "More Small Firms Drop Health Care." *Wall Street Journal*, May 26, 2009, http://online.wsj.com/article/SB124329442612051953.html.

McGuirt, M., et al. "Tennessee Hospital Tells Smokers: You Can't Work Here." ABC News, January 22, 2010, http://abcnews.go.com/Health/QuitToLive/tennessee-hospital-bans-employees-off-job-smoking/story?id=9629201.

Medline Plus. "Heart Failure." http://www.nlm.nih.gov/medlineplus/heartfailure.html.

Merlino, L., et al. "Vitamin D intake is Inversely Associated with Rheumatoid Arthritis: Results from the Iowa Women's Health Study." *Arthritis and Rheumatism* 50 (2004): 72–77.

Mettler, F. A., et al. "Radiologic and Nuclear Medicine Studies in the United States and Worldwide: Frequency, Radiation Dose, and Comparison with Other Radiation Sources—1950–2007." *Radiology* 253 (2009): 520–531.

Middleton, C. "HC Rationing Begins: Younger Breast Cancer Victims Not Important Enough." Liberty Pundits, November 17, 2010, http://libertypundits.net/article/hc-rationing-begins-younger-breast-cancer-victims-not-important-enough/.

Middleton, L., et al. "Promising Strategies for the Prevention of Dementia." *Archives of Neurology* 66 (2009): 1210–1215.

Molinari, N., et al. "The Annual Impact of Seasonal Influenza in the US: Measuring Disease Burden and Costs." *Vaccine* 25 (2007): 5086–96.

Monsivais, P., et al. "The Rising Cost of Low-Energy-Dense Foods." *Journal of the American Dietetic Association* 107 (2007): 2071–2076.

Mozaffarian, D., et al. "Lifestyle Risk Factors and New-Onset Diabetes Mellitus in Older Adults: The Cardiovascular Health Study." *Archives of Internal Medicine* 169 (2009): 798–807.

Mukamal, K., et al. "Alcohol Consumption and Cardiovascular Mortality Among US Adults 1987 to 2002." *Journal of the American College of Cardiology* 55 (2010): 1328–1335.

Mundinger, M., et al. "Primary Care Outcomes in Patients Treated by Nurse Practitioners or Physicians." *Journal of the American Medical Association* 283 (2000): 59–68.

National Cancer Institute. "Obesity and Cancer: Questions and Answers." http://www. cancer.gov/cancertopics/factsheet/Risk/obesity.

———. "Physical Activity and Cancer." http://www.cancer.gov/cancertopics/factsheet/ prevention/physicalactivity.

———. "Prostate-Specific Antigen Test." http://www.cancer.gov/cancertopics/factsheet/ Detection/PSA.

———. "Tumor Markers: Questions and Answers." http://www.cancer.gov/cancertopics/ factsheet/Detection/tumor-markers.

National Highway Traffic Safety Administration. "2006 Motor Vehicle Occupant Protection."http://www.nhtsa.gov/DOT/NHTSA/Traffic%20Injury%20Control/Articles/ Associated%20Files/810654.pdf.

———. "4 Steps for Kids: Seat Belts." http://www.nhtsa.gov/Driving+Safety/Child+Saf ety/4+Steps+for+Kids:+Seat+Belts.

National Institute of Allergy and Infectious Diseases. "Common Cold Overview." http:// www.niaid.nih.gov/topics/commonCold/Pages/overview.aspx.

———. "Common Cold Prevention." http://www.niaid.nih.gov/topics/commonCold/ Pages/prevention.aspx.

National Institute of Diabetes and Digestive and Kidney Diseases. "Am I at Risk for Type 2 Diabetes?" http://diabetes.niddk.nih.gov/dm/pubs/riskfortype2/index.htm#food.

———. "Diabetes Prevention Program." http://diabetes.niddk.nih.gov/dm/pubs/ preventionprogram/.

———. "Diabetes Prevention Program Outcomes Study (DPPOS) Questions & Answers." http://www2.niddk.nih.gov/Research/ClinicalResearch/DPPOS/QA.htm.

———. "Weight and Waist Measurement: Tools for Adults." http://www.win.niddk.nih. gov/publications/tools.htm#circumf.

National Institutes of Health. "Body Mass Index Table 1." http://www.nhlbi.nih.gov/ guidelines/obesity/bmi_tbl.htm.

National Network of Libraries of Medicine. "Health Literacy." http://nnlm.gov/outreach/ consumer/hlthlit.html.

Nichols, G., et al. "Medical Care Costs Among Patients with Established Cardiovascular Disease." *American Journal of Managed Care* 16 (2010): e86–e93.

Nielsen-Bohlman, L., et al. *Health Literacy: A Prescription to End Confusion.* Washington, DC: National Academies Press, 2004.

Nieman, D., et al. "Upper Respiratory Tract Infection Is Reduced in Physically Fit and Active Adults." *British Journal of Sports Medicine.* Online First, November 1, 2010, http://bjsm.bmj.com/content/early/2010/09/30/bjsm.2010.077875.

Oliveira, C., et al. "Toothbrushing, Inflammation, and Risk of Cardiovascular Disease: Results from Scottish Health Survey." *BMJ* 340 (2010): c2451.

Ørtoft, G., et al. "After Conisation of the Cervix, the Perinatal Mortality as a Result of Preterm Delivery Increases in Subsequent Pregnancy." *BJOG: An International Journal of Obstetrics and Gynaecology* 117 (2010): 258–267.

Pallarito, K. "Women Should Ignore New Mammogram Guideline, Ex-NIH Chief Says." HealthDay, http://consumer.healthday.com/Article.asp?AID=633401.

Pan, X., et al. "Effects of Diet and Exercise in Preventing NIDDM in People with Impaired Glucose Tolerance: The Da Qing IGT and Diabetes Study." *Diabetes Care* 20 (1997): 537–544.

Parker, C., et al. "Screening for Prostate Cancer Appears to Work, but at What Cost?" *BJU International* 104 (2009): 290–292.

Partnership for Prescription Assistance. "Questions About the Partnership for Prescription Assistance." http://www.pparx.org/en/questions_about_PPARX.

Patient-Centered Primary Care Collaborative. "The Patient-Centered Medical Home: Quick Reference Guide for Employers." http://www.pcpcc.net/files/pcmhpurchaser summary.pdf.

Payne, J. "Is a Cash-Only or Direct-Pay Medical Practice for You?" *U.S. News & World Report*, January 17, 2009, http://health.usnews.com/health-news/managing-your-healthcare/healthcare/articles/2009/07/17/is-a-cash-only-or-direct-pay-medical-practice-for-you.htm.

Phillips, D., et al. "A July Spike in Fatal Medication Errors: A Possible Effect of New Medical Residents." *Journal of General Internal Medicine* 25 (2010): 774–779.

Pienta, K. "Critical Appraisal of Prostate-specific Antigen in Prostate Cancer Screening: 20 Years Later." *Urology* 73 (2009): S11–S20.

Pitts, S., et al. "National Hospital Ambulatory Medical Care Survey: 2006 Emergency Department Summary." National Health Statistics Reports (2008).

Pullen, P., et al. "Benefits of Yoga for African American Heart Failure Patients." *Medicine and Science in Sports and Exercise* 42 (2009): 651–657.

Redberg, R. "First Physical." *Archives of Internal Medicine* 170 (2010): 583.

Roberts, R. "Seven Reasons Family Doctors Get Sued and How to Reduce Your Risk." *Family Practice Management* 10 (2003): 29–34.

Robinson, J., et al. "Consumer-Driven Health Care: Promise and Performance." *Health Affairs* 28 (2009): 272–281.

Rogers, H., et al. "A Relative Value Unit-Based Cost Comparison of Treatment Modalities for Nonmelanoma Skin Cancer: Effect of the Loss of the Mohs Multiple Surgery Reduction Exemption." *Journal of the American Academy of Dermatology* 61 (2009): 96–103.

Rosell, M., et al. "Dietary Fish and Fish Oil and the Risk of Rheumatoid Arthritis." *Epidemiology* 20 (2009): 896–901.

Sari, N. "Physical Inactivity and Its Impact on Healthcare Utilization." *Health Economics* 18 (2009): 885–901.

Scarmeas, N., et al. "Mediterranean Diet and Risk for Alzheimer's Disease." *Annals of Neurology* 59 (2006): 912–921.

Schroder, F., et al. "Screening and Prostate-cancer Mortality in a Randomized European Study." *New England Journal of Medicine* 360 (2009): 1320–1328.

Sinha, R., et al. "Meat Intake and Mortality." *Archives of Internal Medicine* 169 (2009): 562–571.

Smith, H. "The High Cost of Smoking." MSN Money, http://articles.moneycentral.msn.com/Insurance/InsureYourHealth/HighCostOfSmoking.aspx?page=1.

Smith, R. "Classification and Diagnosis of Patients with Medically Unexplained Symptoms." *Journal of General Internal Medicine* 22 (2007): 685–691.

Smith-Bindman, R. "Radiation Dose Associated with Common Computed Tomography Examinations and the Associated Lifetime Attributable Risk of Cancer." *Archives of Internal Medicine* 169 (2009): 2078–2086.

Sofi, F., et al. "Adherence to Mediterranean Diet and Health Status: Meta-analysis." *BMJ* 337 (2008): a1344.

Sokol, M., et al. "Impact of Medication Adherence on Hospitalization Risk and Healthcare Cost." *Medical Care* 43 (2005): 521–530.

Starfield, B. "Is US Health Really the Best in the World?" *Journal of the American Medical Association* 284 (2000): 483–485.

Sternberg, S. "More Treatment Doesn't Always Mean Better Health." *USA Today*, April 11, 2010, http://www.usatoday.com/news/health/2010-04-12-lessismore12_ST_N.htm.

Studdert, D., et al. "Defensive Medicine Among High-Risk Specialist Physicians in a Volatile Malpractice Environment." *Journal of the American Medical Association* 293 (2005): 2609–2617.

Sugiyama, D., et al. "Impact of Smoking as a Risk Factor for Developing Rheumatoid Arthritis: A Meta-analysis of Observational Studies." *Annals of the Rheumatic Diseases* 69 (2010): 70–81.

Sun, Q., et al. "White Rice, Brown Rice, and Risk of Type 2 Diabetes in US Men and Women." *Archives of Internal Medicine* 170 (2010): 961–969.

Surveillance Epidemiology and End Results. "SEER Stat Fact Sheets: Breast." http://seer.cancer.gov/statfacts/html/breast.html.

———. "Melanoma of the Skin." http://seer.cancer.gov/statfacts/html/melan.html.

———. "SEER Stat Fact Sheets: Oral Cavity and Pharynx." http://seer.cancer.gov/statfacts/html/oralcav.html.

Tang L., et al. "Consumption of Raw Cruciferous Vegetables Is Inversely Associated with Bladder Cancer Risk." *Cancer Epidemiology, Biomarkers & Prevention* 17 (2008): 938–944.

Taylor, D., et al. "Population-Based Family History–Specific Risks for Colorectal Cancer: A Constellation Approach." *Gastroenterology* 138 (2010): 877–885.

Thompson, P., et al. "Exercise and Physical Activity in the Prevention and Treatment of Atherosclerotic Cardiovascular Disease." *Circulation* 107 (2003): 3109–3116.

Thorpe, K., et al. "Differences in Disease Prevalence as a Source of the U.S.-European Health Care Spending Gap." *Health Affairs* 26 (2007): 678–686.

Truffer, C., et al. "Health Spending Projections Through 2019: The Recession's Impact Continues." *Health Affairs* 29 (2010): 522–529.

University of Maryland Medical Center. "Infertility in Men— Risk Factors." http://www. umm.edu/patiented/articles/how_do_sperm_abnormalities_contribute_male_infertility _000067_3.htm.

Urquhart, D., et al. "Factors that May Mediate the Relationship Between Physical Activity and the Risk for Developing Knee Osteoarthritis." *Arthritis Research & Therapy* 10:208. Epub February 4, 2008.

U.S. Census Bureau. "Projected Population of the United States, by Age and Sex: 2000 to 2050." http://www.census.gov/population/www/projections/usinterimproj/natpro jtab02a.pdf

U.S. Central Intelligence Agency. "Country Comparison: Infant Mortality Rate." https:// www.cia.gov/library/publications/the-world-factbook/rankorder/2091rank.html.

———. "Country Comparison: Life Expectancy at Birth." https://www.cia.gov/library/ publications/the-world-factbook/rankorder/2102rank.html.

U.S. Consumer Product Safety Commission. "Childproofing Your Home." http://www. cpsc.gov/cpscpub/pubs/252.pdf.

U.S. Department of Health and Human Services. "Polycystic Ovary Syndrome (PCOS)." http://www.nichd.nih.gov/publications/pubs/upload/PCOS_booklet.pdf.

———. "Polycystic Ovary Syndrome (PCOS) Frequently Asked Questions." http://www. womenshealth.gov/faq/polycystic-ovary-syndrome.cfm.

U.S. Department of Labor. "Occupational Outlook Handbook, 2010–11 Edition: Physician Assistants." http://www.bls.gov/oco/ocos081.htm.

———. "Occupational Outlook Handbook, 2010–11 Edition: Physicians and Surgeons." http://www.bls.gov/oco/ocos074.htm.

U.S. Equal Employment Opportunity Commission. "Questions and Answers About Cancer in the Workplace and the Americans with Disabilities Act (ADA)." http:// www.eeoc.gov/facts/cancer.html.

U.S. Food and Drug Administration. "Facts About Generic Drugs." http://www.fda.gov/ Drugs/EmergencyPreparedness/BioterrorismandDrugPreparedness/ucm134010.htm.

———. "Facts and Myths About Generic Drugs." http://www.fda.gov/Drugs/Resources ForYou/Consumers/BuyingUsingMedicineSafely/UnderstandingGenericDrugs/ ucm167991.htm.

———. "Generic Drugs: Questions and Answers." http://www.fda.gov/Drugs/Resources ForYou/Consumers/QuestionsAnswers/ucm100100.htm.

U.S. Preventive Services Task Force. "Screening for Abdominal Aortic Aneurysm." http:// www.uspreventiveservicestaskforce.org/uspstf/uspsaneu.htm.

———. "Screening for Breast Cancer." http://www.uspreventiveservicestaskforce.org/ uspstf/uspsbrca.htm.

———. "Screening for Cervical Cancer." http://www.uspreventiveservicestaskforce.org/ uspstf/uspscerv.htm.

———. "Screening for Colorectal Cancer." http://www.uspreventiveservicestaskforce. org/uspstf/uspscolo.htm.

———. "Screening for Coronary Heart Disease." http://www.uspreventiveservicestask force.org/uspstf/uspsacad.htm.

———. "Screening for Osteoporosis." http://www.uspreventiveservicestaskforce.org/ uspstf/uspsoste.htm.

———. "Screening for Prostate Cancer." http://www.uspreventiveservicestaskforce.org/ uspstf/uspsprca.htm.

Vernon, J., et al. "Low Health Literacy: Implications for National Health Policy." National Patient Safety Foundation. http://npsf.org/askme3/pdfs/Case_Report_10_07.pdf.

Viscusi, W., et al. "The Mortality Cost to Smokers." *Journal of Health Economics* 27 (2008): 943–958.

Wassertheil-Smoller, S., et al. "Depression and Cardiovascular Sequelae in Postmeno-pausal Women." *Archives of Internal Medicine* 164 (2004): 289–298.

Weaver, K., et al. "Forgoing Medical Care Because of Cost." *Cancer* 116 (2010): 3493–3504.

Weinstein, S. "The Cost of Defensive Medicine." American Academy of Orthopaedic Surgeons/American Association of Orthopaedic Surgeons. http://www.aaos.org/news/aaosnow/nov08/managing7.asp.

Welch, H., et al. "Prostate Cancer Diagnosis and Treatment After Introduction of Pros-tate-Specific Antigen Screening: 1986–2005." *Journal of the National Cancer Institute* 101 (2009): 1325–1329.

Weyer, C., et al. "Insulin Action and Insulinemia Are Closely Related to the Fasting Complement C3, but Not Acylation Stimulating Protein Concentration." *Diabetes Care* 23 (2000): 779–785.

The White House. "Press Briefing by Dr. Connie Mariano on the President's Annual Medical Check-up." http://clinton5.nara.gov/library/hot_briefings/January_12_2001. html.

Windustry. "How Much Do Wind Turbines Cost?" http://www.windustry.org/how-much-do-wind-turbines-cost.

Winterstein, A., et al. "Evaluation of Consumer Medication Information Dispensed in Retail Pharmacies." *Archives of Internal Medicine* 170 (2010): 1317–1324.

Wolfe, F., et al. "Out-of-Pocket Expenses and Their Burden in Patients with Rheumatoid Arthritis." *Arthritis & Rheumatism* 61 (2009): 1563–1570.

Wolin, K., et al. "Physical Activity and Colon Cancer Prevention: A Meta-Analysis." *British Journal of Cancer* 100 (2009): 611–616.

Wright, J. "Overshooting Obama's Health." NPR, http://www.npr.org/templates/story/story.php?storyId=124279916.

Yankaskas, B., et al. "Performance of First Mammography Examination in Women Younger than 40 Years." *Journal of the National Cancer Institute* 102 (2010): 692–701.

Yin, M., et al. "Prevalence of Incidental Prostate Cancer in the General Population: A Study of Healthy Organ Donors." *Journal of Urology* 179 (2008): 892–895.

Index

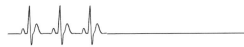

About the Authors

Cindy Haines, M.D., is a board-certified family physician and faculty member in the Department of Family and Community Medicine at the Saint Louis University School of Medicine. She is the chief medical officer of HealthDay, a consumer news service that provides daily health news to thousands of internet and intranet sites including Yahoo.com, MedlinePlus, MSN.com, and a wide variety of hospital sites.

Dr. Haines is also managing editor of Physician's Briefing, HealthDay's news wire service for healthcare professionals. As the host of HealthDay TV, her daily news reports reach millions of viewers each month. Dr. Haines is also a featured medical editor and/or medical writer on a variety of health information websites. The New Prescription is her first book.

Dr. Haines is a member of several professional organizations, including the American Medical Association and the American Diabetes Association. She served as president of the Saint Louis Academy of Family Physicians in 2010, is currently serving as past president (2011), and is a diplomat of the American Academy of Family Physicians. She is also a member of the international Mensa society.

She lives with her husband, Will, and their two children, Isabella (Elle) and Wm. Dennison, in her hometown of St. Louis, Missouri.

Eric Metcalf is a health writer, author, and radio commentator based in Indianapolis. He has coauthored or contributed to more than a dozen health and fitness books, and his work has appeared in national magazines and major health websites.